SKIN SECRETS

SKIN SECRETS

A Complete Guide
to Skin Care
for the Entire Family

JOSEPH P. BARK, M.D.

McGraw-Hill Book Company

New York   St. Louis   San Francisco   Auckland   Bogotá
Hamburg   Johannesburg   London   Madrid
Mexico   Milan   Montreal   New Delhi   Panama
Paris   São Paulo   Singapore   Sydney   Tokyo   Toronto

This book is not intended to replace the services of a physician. Any application of the recommendations set forth in the following pages is at the reader's discretion. The reader should consult with his or her own physician concerning the recommendations made in this book.

1 2 3 4 5 6 7 8 9 DOCDOC 8 7

ISBN 0-07-003671-3

LIBRARY OF CONGRESS CATALOGING IN PUBLICATION DATA

Bark, Joseph P.
   Skin secrets.
   1. Skin—Care and hygiene.   2. Dermatology—Popular
works.   I. Title.
RL87.B35   1987   616.5   86-18010
ISBN 0-07-003671-3

BOOK DESIGN BY PATRICE FODERO
EDITING SUPERVISOR: MARGERY LUHRS

To Mom—The Heart
To Glenn—The Spark
To Bob Braun—The Fire
To Lin—The Love

Contents

Acknowledgments   ix

Preface   xi

Chapter 1:   O.S.I.G.U.W.A.D. (Okay, So I Give Up.
              What's a Dermatologist?)   1

Chapter 2:   Diaper Rash—The Bane of Babies'
              Bottoms   5

Chapter 3:   Birthmarks   11

Chapter 4:   Skin Infections—Warts, Impetigo, and
              Other Common Skin Problems   21

Chapter 5:   Eczema—How to Put Out the Fire on
              Your Child's Skin   37

Chapter 6:   Poison Ivy—Leave These Leaves Alone!   43

Chapter 7:   The War Against Acne—A Struggle to
              Save Face   49

Chapter 8:   Restoring Acne-Scarred Skin   81

Chapter 9:   Nonacne Problems of the Young   93

Chapter 10: Hair—Either Famine or Feast   111

Chapter 11: Nothing Stops Dandruff Like a Dark Blue
                 Suit!   139

Chapter 12: Her Skin   145

Chapter 13: His Skin   179

Chapter 14: Black Skin—Some Good News and Some
                 Bad News   189

Chapter 15: Fingernails—Proper Care of Our "First
                 Tools"   197

Chapter 16: Beating Psoriasis—How to Live Without
                 Leaving a Trail of Scales   203

Chapter 17: Fry Now, Pay Later—Sun Cancers,
                 Melanomas, and Moles   223

Chapter 18: Herpes—The New Leprosy   259

Chapter 19: Winter Itch—The Problems of Dry Skin   271

Chapter 20: New Wrinkles on Aging Skin   279

Chapter 21: The Real Skin Secret Is You!   305

                 Index   309

Acknowledgments

I owe a lot to a lot of people who helped in the preparation of this book. Thanks go to all our friends who tolerated my disappearing act on many, many vacations, when I stole off with my pencil and pad, or word processor, and stack of mail from the *Braun & Company* TV show to generate the questions and answers you'll read here.

My thanks go to Dr. Glenn Marsh, who first aroused the spark of interest in skin medicine and who provided so many of the skin secrets I learned myself in the early days of my career. That spark has grown into a roaring fire that has led to a career of providing public medical information as much as dermatology. It's his respect for patients as people that has always made his approach to dermatology special.

I'm grateful to Jim Witham, my writing coach, who convinced me I could make my thoughts understandable, readable, and interesting, with a lot of good ideas, sweat, and an unlimited number of rewrites.

And a special thanks goes to Kathy J. Adair, whose nimble fingers and skill with an IBM Displaywriter have condensed a ten-year job into five. She has patiently tolerated more rewrites and deadlines than a normal person encounters in a lifetime. Without her this book would still be a fervent wish.

To Peggy Blair Richards and my other office staff who have read parts of the manuscript and offered constructive advice, my heartfelt thanks.

Preface

Sometime late in my third year at the University of Kentucky College of Medicine I was working in the neonatal intensive care unit. As I was trying to insert a small butterfly needle into a scalp vein of an infant, a fellow in a bright sport coat walked leisurely in to the neonatal unit, put on a sterile gown, and came into the "baby brig" as we called it. He stepped up to my side and announced, "I'm Marsh in dermatology. Is the Saunders baby here?"

"Yes," I said, pointing to the next incubator, "That's him over there." Dr. Glenn Marsh strolled over and very gently picked up a tiny leg with a bulbous, red spot on the thigh. I remembered seeing it on rounds earlier in the day.

"Hemangioma," he said. "No sweat!"

"You mean you can fix it?" I asked, as I pulled out my second try at the scalp vein.

Marsh glanced over his shoulder and said, "God'll fix that one, Doctor Bark," glancing at my name tag. "Most of them go away without any treatment at all."

"Fascinating!" I said, as I prepared to stick my diminutive patient again. "We thought he'd be in for long hours under the knife!"

"Nope. They fade beautifully almost every time! You ought to think about dermatology. I think you'd find it *very* interesting!" And, in fact, the dermatology elective I took in Dr. Marsh's private office the next year introduced me to my career of answering questions about the skin.

Later, in my residency in dermatology, I found myself faced with a very quizzical look on a patient named John with white spots on his face. I was explaining to John that he had a very common problem of middle age. It was sebaceous hyperplasia. I went on to explain that sometimes the sebaceous glands of the face underwent hypertrophy during the aging process.

With my every word John's face showed more and more confusion, until finally he said, "Listen Doctor, have you been talking to *me* for the last five minutes? If so," he said, "you'd better give me a few years to go to medical school before you continue this explanation. Then I *might* understand it!"

I decided then and there to launch a campaign to make medicine more easily understandable to those who matter the most: my patients.

Since then I've found that one of the greatest thrills in medicine is the thanks of a patient who has had a problem explained in words that can be understood. It seems that we doctors just don't seem to take the time to do that anymore. I wish all doctors would realize that "enlarged oil glands accompanying middle age" sounds infinitely better than "hyperplastic pilosebaceous follicles."

So it has become a hobby for me, you see, a sort of constant challenge, to explain things to my patients in words they'll understand.

I don't always succeed. For instance, a young woman named Mary came to me one day with a vaginal yeast infection and a very itchy discharge. After her examination I was interested to find out if she and her husband were ping-ponging this infectious yeast back and forth, so I asked her, "Is your husband circumcised?" A quizzical look followed. So, not wanting to give her more time to be embarrassed, I further questioned and explained, "Well, does he have a foreskin on his penis?" Mary mumbled a terse word or two I could not hear. We both squirmed a little, and I realized I was in trouble.

I decided I could either drop the subject and miss a possible source of contagion (along with the possible embarrassment), or I could pursue it further. Unfortunately, I pursued it. I next held up a thumb as if to represent a penis and slowly encircled it with my index finger as if to demonstrate where a foreskin might be located. "Does he have a *foreskin* on his *penis*?" I asked, more emphatically.

Mary, growing livid with my pursuit of the subject, glowered straight at me and said, "Doctor, I just do not know!"

I decided it was time to break off the inquiry. I felt sure if he had that infection under his foreskin that he would eventually have found his way to a physician for treatment. Sometimes the doctor can't win no matter what words are used.

You can see that medical explanations can quickly get out of hand. But I've tried to break down the medical terminology and vital dermatologic information in this book into terms which are understandable to those outside the medical community. Realize, though, that in a single volume I can really only attack the most prevalent problems involved in dermatologic care.

Since the skin is the largest and most visible of all the body's organs, the science of dermatology is one of the oldest of all medical sciences.

In the last fifty years, dermatology has acquired a great deal of respect from the general medical community for dealing with a vast array of cutaneous illnesses unknown to ordinary physicians during their medical training.

Because I have spent my professional career answering questions, even traveling all over the country speaking about skin care, I felt patients' questions would be a very natural source of material for *Skin Secrets*. So at the behest of Bob Braun, host of a widely acclaimed and very successful talk show in the Midwest, I have patterned the book around these questions.

I have tried wherever possible to highlight new, exciting, or maximally important information in "Dermalert" blocks. You'll see them scattered throughout the book as an aid in picking up the real "pearls" of the subject. My fervent thanks go to the thousands of patients who have contributed most of the questions included in this book.

1

O.S.I.G.U.W.A.D.?*

Everyone knows a barometer can predict weather changes days in advance, but few realize that the skin, as the body's barometer, can predict health and illness far in advance. However, these signs are often very subtle, requiring the trained eye and awareness of one who has devoted a lifetime to the art of cutaneous diagnosis—the dermatologist.

DERMALERT

Skin problems can herald the onset of internal problems. Your dermatologist uses the skin as a window on your body's internal mechanisms. Don't fail to consult your dermatologist if something unusual is happening.

Take Paul, for instance, an elderly patient sent to me by another physician for a very painful outbreak of shingles. We'll talk more

*Okay, So I Give Up. What's A Dermatologist?

about shingles later, but basically it's a virus infection caused by reactivation of the chicken pox virus. But Paul's eruption was quite different. He had the typical blisters of the disease, but they had spread outside the normal streaklike shingles distribution.

As we talked, I learned that he had lost fifteen pounds in the last forty-five days unintentionally. A physical exam and chest x-ray revealed that Paul had Hodgkin's disease, a type of cancer of the lymph nodes. His skin had warned us that something was wrong internally. He's doing well now on chemotherapy and his shingles are, of course, gone.

Certainly shingles does not always indicate a serious disease, but it's an example of the type of problem dermatologists solve daily for their patients and referring physicians. Let's look at some of the many general questions patients have about dermatology and skin doctors.

Your Skin Doctor

Q: Are dermatologists *real* doctors, too? The reason I asked is that my skin doctor wouldn't treat my sore throat one time. What, exactly, does it take to become a dermatologist?

A: Dermatologists are indeed medical doctors or doctors of osteopathy as well. They've completed four years of medical school to get their medical degree, a year of internship, and three years of residency.

But most dermatologists are pretty strict at sticking to the specialty for which we're trained—skin medicine. That's not to say that, in an emergency, we wouldn't treat you for something else, but as a rule, your family doctor should handle your sore throat and other general medical problems.

Q: When are skin problems severe enough to warrant seeing a dermatologist?

A: If a problem can be seen or felt, it can be initially evaluated by a dermatologist. That does not mean that all such problems can be handled by the dermatologist, but it's certainly an excellent starting point if you are concerned about any skin spot or symptom. Itching, for instance, which is usually a reaction to external irritants, can also be a sign of diabetes and many other internal diseases, such as hidden malignancies and infections.

DERMALERT

The time to see a dermatologist about a skin problem is as soon as you notice one.

Q: What can I expect from my dermatologist?

A: Your dermatologist, like any other physician, will establish basic information about your background through the use of your medical record. He or she will question you about the history of your problem, including significant past and social history, and will perform an examination of the skin and other systems pertinent to your complaint.

To clarify the diagnosis of difficult rashes, many dermatologists are equipped to perform laboratory tests such as fungus cultures and various other stains and microscopic preparations right in their offices.

Dermatology is a peculiarly mixed specialty, having medical and surgical modes. Almost every dermatologist does minor surgery, and many do dermabrasions, minor cosmetic surgery, and minor plastic surgical procedures.

Q: How much does it cost?

A: I hate to hedge on the question of costs. However, dermatologic costs are found to vary greatly among practitioners and more so among various areas of the country where fee schedules have been established. A guesstimate, however, is that initial office fees for a dermatologist will run in the $25 to $50 bracket; surgical charges, injections, and medications will add to this figure.

I suggest to anyone who has questions about charges that they talk to their doctor frankly about this *before* procedures are done or medication given.

Q: Are prescription medicines (both internal and topical) more beneficial than over-the-counter preparations?

A: In general they are, because over-the-counter medicine companies cannot make their medicines strong enough to do as much good because of the risk of side effects. The fact that a medicine is dispensed by prescription means that there are certain risks or side effects which must be weighed against the benefits of using the medicine to clear a specific skin problem. This judgment is made by the physician who then has the license to write the prescription, and accepts responsibility for doing so.

So if you have used an over-the-counter medicine to treat a specific skin problem and it is not working, see a dermatologist for further guidance and possibly prescription medicines.

DERMALERT

As a general rule prescription medicines are more effective than over-the-counter medicines.

Where to Go for Help

If you want information about certain topics not mentioned in this book, consult your dermatologist. Ask your dermatologist for information sheets or handouts concerning your skin disease or condition. You can then refer to them for salient treatment points when you wish to recall them later. Call your dermatologist or write to:

The American Academy of Dermatology
820 Davis Street
P.O. Box 271
Evanston, Illinois 60201

2

Diaper Rash—The Bane of Babies' Bottoms

Each time a newborn baby is delivered, an amazing counting process begins. Every parent wants to make sure that his or her baby came off the assembly line with all its parts. After checking the number of fingers and toes, new parents then begin to inspect that fantastic material covering them, skin. It's an examination process that will proceed for the rest of the child's life.

Isn't it incredible that in just nine short months the embryonic skin develops every one of the thousands of structures within it that are present in adult skin—oil glands, hair, hair muscles, nerves, blood vessels, sweat glands—everything! And it all works. A newborn's skin is already such a fantastic air-conditioning unit that babies can easily grow cold because of its efficient heat transfer. In fact, that's why babies wear stocking caps—their head skin comprises a much greater proportion of their total body skin than does the head skin of an adult.

Most of us manage our own skins pretty well, but we panic when it comes time to tend the delicate skin of the newborn. The difference is that we're not struggling to survive in a totally new, completely alien atmosphere, replete with threats of yeast in diapers, irritation from soaps and lotions, and a thousand other threats every day.

Every parent needs to know the problems of infant skin—its infections, allergies, and even birthmarks. Let's start with some of the most commonly asked questions about diaper rash.

Diaper Rash

Q: No matter what I do, my baby keeps getting horrible reddish diaper rashes. I cannot understand it, because I use the best disposable diapers. Even the new elastic-legged ones haven't helped. What's your solution?

A: It's always been amazing how little is understood by the general medical community (let alone parents) about what causes diaper rash. The diaper dilemma was solved for me by a few simple words from one of the most respected pediatricians ever known, the late Dr. Warren Wheeler of the University of Kentucky. While I was doing an admission physical exam on a baby one day, Dr. Wheeler noticed that my patient's groin was as red as a fire truck. He ambled over to the baby's bed with his quick little hopping step, put his hands on his hips, and peered at my patient with his big bespectacled eyes as I went through the physical exam (quite nervously, under the gaze of the department chairman). Finally he blurted out excitedly, "Doctor, why do you think that little peanut has that diaper rash?"

"Well, judging by my lecture notes, I'd say that it's probably ammonia, Dr. Wheeler."

"No, I mean why does he have a *diaper* rash? My point, Dr. Bark, is that this little pumpkin probably has a diaper rash because he's wearing a diaper. Leave that diaper off, and you'll cure him, sure as shootin'!" He walked off briskly, smiling to himself that he had given yet another med student a tip that would serve him a lifetime.

That very simple fact, which should be obvious to every physician, mother, and father concerned with diaper rash, often completely escapes their minds. Since those days in medical school, I've successfully treated hundreds of cases of diaper rash just by having the parents keep the child out of diapers whenever possible.

DERMALERT

Diapers cause diaper *rash*!

Just as important, however, since most parents will not avoid diapers altogether because of the mess involved, is the use of the right *type* of diaper. Our modern, disposable, throwaway age has led us to believe that disposable diapers are the final answer to baby care. The simple and unavoidable truth of infancy is "what eats, excretes," and the problem of diaper rash is avoidable with the proper "care and maintenance" of your kid's south side.

This means using the old-fashioned cotton diapers instead of the disposable type. Yes, I know this book is slamming shut all across the nation, but for any kid who has a tendency toward diaper dermatitis, this tip is crucial to prevention. Let me explain further about the reasoning behind the use of cloth diapers. For years we have been looking after the convenience and ease of the parents at the expense of the babies who have to wear disposable diapers. The problem grew even worse when the plastic covering was invented for the paper diaper. The plastic keeps the *parent* away from the wetness, not the child!

We'd all like to think that every mother changes her baby's diapers as soon as they are wet, but in practice we know the system is less than perfect and the baby often does sit in urine for some time before changing, even in the most meticulous of families. The crucial question is who sits in the wet urine? You guessed it! It's the baby in that disposable diaper with the plastic outer covering. The humidity in there is 100 percent. This makes a magnificent culture medium for the growth of yeast, which is normally found in a baby's diaper area. This yeast then grows and invades the tender skin of your baby's bottom, making a red, itchy, scaly, sometimes weeping and bleeding irritation of the skin.

The problem has been greatly compounded over the last few years with the advent of disposable diapers with elastic around the leg band areas so that no moisture can escape.

DERMALERT

The bane of babies' bottoms is the disposable plastic-covered diaper. Some babies can be treated for diaper rash just by leaving the diaper off whenever possible and by switching to soft cloth diapers when necessary.

Another problem with the diaper area is the use of thick ointments on a baby as a more or less continuous form of "protection" of the tender groin areas. Babies have been brought in to my office so thickly coated with ointment and baby powder that it has taken half an hour to scrub all the goo from the skin so that I could see the rash!

If you want to cleanse your baby's bottom, do it with a nice *mild* soap like Dove, and use a *mild* antiyeast, drying powder like Caldesene. Never use ointments unless your doctor prescribes them.

DERMALERT

Don't put heavy ointments on your baby's bottom. These only cover up the diaper rash and may actually worsen it.

So the "bottom" line on diaper dermatitis is this: use paper disposable diapers judiciously (or not at all), if your baby has any tendency toward diaper rash. Keep it simple. Clean the child with a mild soap and maybe you won't have your neighbors and parents asking if your child is really a little lobster.

Topicals for Infants

Q: My pediatrician told me when I delivered my child not to put powder or oil on his skin. Do you agree, and if so, why is it not good? Also, what do you think about cornstarch powders? Do you think the new premoistened paper wipes are okay to use at diaper changes?

A: Early in dermatology training, we are told to listen carefully to pediatricians when they make comments about the skin.
Why? Because pediatricians get to see so *much* skin and so *many*
skin problems, that they become excellent dermatologists over the
years. In your case, I would have to agree that unless your child
has a problem, there is no real need to put baby oil on his skin.
If your child has a dry, scaly skin rash, it is certainly harmless to
try baby oil as a type of moisturizer for a while, and I think most
of us in dermatology, and certainly most mothers and pediatricians, would agree that baby powder is fairly harmless and a very
pleasant substance to use. I can remember times when I was a
child getting out of a bathtub, drying well, and then being doused
thoroughly with baby powder. It always felt very good and never
caused any problem. Use it if you like.

If you ever have the opportunity to look at baby powder under
a microscope you will see that the talc in the powder looks like
tiny jagged pieces of glass under magnification. It's really hard
to imagine how such a substance could be put on soft baby skin
without being irritating! But in fact, the jagged edges of the talc
flakes must be compensated for by the incredible smoothness and
flatness of the tiny plates of powder. The theory is that even
though the edges are somewhat jagged, the flakes actually do
glide over one another very smoothly.

I don't think much of cornstarch powders. Cornstarch has been
known to support yeast growth, which, as you already know, is
a chronic source of diaper rash and irritation. Therefore, if you
want a good powder, use Caldesene. It's available in a pink can
in the baby section of drugstores. This agent has talc, but it also
has an antiyeast substance which can help prevent diaper rash in
your child.

DERMALERT

Cornstarch may promote yeast growth on your baby.
Save it for your kitchen.

Premoistened paper wipes are safe to use at diaper changes provided the infant shows no allergic reaction to them. (However,
I've never known anyone to encounter such problems.)

3

Birthmarks

A birthmark is a spot on the skin which is present on the person's day of birth. There are many types of birthmarks, and they are often lifelong problems.

Why is it that some of us are born with faultless, unsmudged skin, and others are born with birthmarks? We just don't know. We do know that some types of moles are heritable, but we have very little information on the origins of other types.

Chance? Genetics? Some developmental accident? Drugs? Toxins? Maybe all or none. A study in *Clinical Pediatrics* (August 1978) showed that 21 percent of children with hemangiomas (the red type) had a definite family history of them. That's much higher than the population in general and does indeed indicate that heredity plays some part in their development.

Some birthmarks represent serious problems, occasionally even life-threatening ones; others are lifelong stains which can affect every facet of one's life. Let's consider the various types separately.

Q: When my son was about one month old I noticed a small brown flat spot near his left eye. Should I have it examined by a dermatologist? Also, is it possible it could have been caused by silver nitrate put in his eyes at birth? Finally, why is it that this mark did not appear until he was one month old?

A: There is some possibility that this spot is a café au lait spot (French for "coffee with milk"; these spots actually do have this shading). Have your child examined by a dermatologist. The child may have other skin conditions and even internal problems related to the skin spot which should be discussed with your dermatologist.

It was not the silver nitrate which caused this discoloration. Silver nitrate discoloration is superficial, does not usually occur with the eyedrops, and occurs within hours of the exposure, not months.

I can't adequately explain why this mark appeared at one month of age. Many of the pigmented spots do gradually darken during infancy and childhood, however.

Note that if your child does have a café au lait spot, it can be masked much more easily than some of the darker spots we will talk about in succeeding questions.

DERMALERT

Flat brown spots on children should be examined by your dermatologist because these flat spots can be an indicator of other skin diseases. Some are associated with serious health problems which need to be treated early.

Hairy Birthmarks

Q: I am 24 years old and have had a raised, hairy mole since birth. I have heard that these spots occasionally turn into skin cancers. Do my chances of getting cancer in the raised mole increase the longer it remains? Does removal require surgery in the hospital or can it be done in a doctor's office? Who does it, a dermatologist?

A: Brown, raised, hairy moles represent a completely different type of birthmark. For years it was thought that these moles were benign and could be left alone because they never turned into skin cancers. The exception to this was the large "bathing trunk nevus" which covered widespread areas on the back in the the bathing suit area. These often developed into a very serious life-threatening form of skin cancer called *malignant melanoma*. One study, in the 1977 *Scandinavian Journal of Plastic and Reconstructive Surgery*, indicates that 5 percent of them turn into fatal melanomas. I will have more to say about malignant melanoma in a later chapter.

In the wake of years of observation by skin cancer experts, dermatologists have come to the conclusion that these moles, thought so long to be no problem to the children who have them, should now be removed. It is estimated that some 7 to 17 percent of them, if they are dark brown and were present on the day of the child's birth, will turn into malignant melanoma at some time during the child's life. Usually this malignant degeneration occurs before the late teens, though it can occur at any time.

So dermatologists who study these *congenital melanocytic nevi*, as they are called, now suggest that early removal is the best possible course. In the 1977 Scandinavian study, every child whose mole turned to melanoma died. Naturally, it is a huge task for a surgeon to remove very large lesions from the back and the buttocks. But it should and can be done with the advice and help of a plastic surgeon.

If the moles are small, they can easily be taken off and closed primarily, that is, with a simple line of stitches, right in the doctor's office. However, the larger lesions sometimes require removal in strips and often may require skin grafts to cover the defect. Plastic surgeons usually do the larger mole removals, but some dermatologists (who are also dermatologic surgeons) can do this procedure.

DERMALERT

Seven to 17 percent of dark brown, hairy moles present since birth can turn into a deadly skin cancer. Have your dermatologist check *any* pigmented spot on your child.

Port-Wine Stains

The story of red birthmarks is one of the saddest chapters in dermatologic history. The conventional term for this type of spot is *port-wine stain* (PWS), or *nevus flammeus*. The term originated in the 1800s when the town of O Porto shipped dark red wine to England. In England, physicians noticed that spills of this port wine on tablecloths looked like the color of the nevus flammeus.

Today, while we still don't know the cause of PWS spots, we do know some things which should be done for them, and some things which should not be done.

Port-wine stains are collections of dilated, or widely opened, superficial blood veins, or capillaries, which often appear at birth or a few months thereafter. They are a lot darker and redder than the "salmon patch," which is a lighter birthmark usually over the back, upper neck, and glabellar area of the forehead (the small triangle over the nasal bridge area). Port-wine stains usually start out as slightly pink spots which get slowly redder through childhood and darken into a deep wine red in adolescence and early adulthood. They actually turn frankly purple and bumpy in middle and old age. They can sometimes cover the entire length of the leg or occasionally half the body.

Sometimes these spots can cause massive swelling of the tissues in the areas occupied by the lesions. This can result in enlargement of the bones and body structures below these spots.

Q: I was born with a red birthmark on the upper right side of my face. My mother accounted for this by telling me that, while she was pregnant, a neighbor's house caught fire. She says she put her hand to the right side of her face in fear and terror, and that's what caused my mark. What do you think?

A: There's no way at all that the fire tragedy had anything to do with your spot.

Q: I have a huge reddish birthmark on my leg. I often sit and dream what it would be like to have two nice, white legs. My family tells me I should not worry about it, but I can't help it; it's just awful and ugly. Please, if you have any suggestions, let me know. Even if there's nothing that can be done, at least I'll know I have tried.

A: There have been hundreds of different treatments tried for PWS throughout the history of medicine. For years small ones were cut off and the defect was sewn shut, producing a scar of variable size and length. This works well for small spots if the patient can tolerate the scar that results, but for large spots, and for those spots which involve vital structures such as the eyelid, there is no way to do this surgery without leaving a mark which looks much worse than the PWS. Cryosurgery (freezing) has been tried with very little success, and so has tattooing the lesions with flesh-colored ink. This latter can occasionally dull the tone of the redness, but the look is usually unsatisfactory.

However, over the last ten years a "new light" has appeared on the horizon for those with PWS. That light is the argon laser. This is truly one of the great success stories in medicine, since the technique works best in those lesions which are the worst—purple, dark, nodular marks on the face.

Pioneered by dermatologist Dr. Leon Goldman of the University of Cincinnati and followed up by the highly skilled Laser Treatment Unit of Beth-Israel Hospital in Boston, Massachusetts, laser therapy means great relief from a stigma which can literally destroy one's life.

This therapy is most effective for those who are over 17 years old and who have deep red to purple and even nodular lesions. Regrettably it does not work as well in the very young and/or in those with pink or light red lesions. This is unfortunate for the young because the lightening of these spots could result in a much more relaxed and successful childhood.

Laser treatment for PWS, however, is difficult and somewhat painful. Usually more than one treatment is required, and there is no guarantee that the mark will be completely erased. Frankly, complete removal is often not possible. The laser surgeon's aim is to decrease the defect as much as possible. The laser treatments *can* involve scarring. However, this is very infrequent and usually occurs in specific areas of the head and neck.

The treatment even works on eyelids, a fact which makes it the most effective and advanced form of spot removal for this location.

If you have a port-wine stain which is annoying or causing significant problems for you, discuss it with your dermatologist and ask for a referral to a center for laser treatment. Many dermatologists in private practice are now highly skilled in the use of the laser.

DERMALERT

> Port-wine stains are large red birthmarks that may be significantly helped by various types of laser surgery. This surgery is being performed daily in this country, and if you, your child, or a relative has a port-wine stain, you should consider looking into this excellent new therapy.

PWS patients should keep in mind, however, that their skin markings may be with them throughout life. They should also keep in mind that their friends will accept them because they *are* their friends. Remember, too, that even if the marks cannot be removed, there are ways to disguise them.

The Covermark System

Lydia O'Leary designed the Covermark makeup system in the late 1930s to be used over port-wine stains. It's so dramatically effective in PWS lesions that dermatologists themselves sometimes find it nearly undetectable. I first saw the Covermark system demonstrated at an American Academy of Dermatology meeting several years ago. A very pleasant lady was showing all the techniques used for covering port-wine stains and other lesions. She showed a picture of a young woman who somehow looked quite familiar to me but had an incredible dark purple port-wine stain covering half her face. In the next picture, this same lady's face was completely "free" of this gigantic deforming lesion. It was then that I realized where I had seen the lady in this picture. It was a picture of the lady *showing* the very pictures we were looking at! Standing in front of me was the same lady some ten years older than she was in the picture but wearing her Covermark cosmetics, so that I had not even suspected she had the PWS problem.

She went on to demonstrate the various techniques for effectively covering all types of skin blemishes, including unsightly enlarged veins on the legs. Since that time I have prescribed Covermark cosmetics for blemishes of every shape, size, and description. The system has worked well for nearly all these patients.

The Lydia O'Leary Covermark office is now at:

1 Anderson Avenue
Moonachie, New Jersey 07074
(201) 460-7713

You may contact them for brochures regarding the availability of Covermark cosmetics and their other products in your area. They may be tough to find, but they are certainly worth the trouble.

Strawberry Marks

Q: I have a daughter who was born with a strawberry mark between her eyebrows. I was told it would vanish, but it hasn't. It has dispersed somewhat and is not highly noticeable, but she is extremely self-conscious of it despite being only 5 years old. We never mention it in front of her, and she wears bangs to cover it. I frequently find her examining it closely in mirrors, particularly in department stores, where the lighting is much stronger than at home. Is there any safe and effective way to permanently remove this birthmark?

A: If your daughter's mark is truly a strawberry birthmark, it's a small collection of abnormally growing blood vessels which usually increase in size slightly during the first year or so of life. After this time it will usually become stable or start to regress.

To remember best the natural course of a strawberry birthmark, you should remember the numbers 5, 7, and 9. The 5 stands for the fact that 50 percent of these lesions are gone completely by the age of 5, 70 percent are usually gone by the age of 7, and 90 percent are gone by the age of 9. While this does not hold as a hard and fast rule by any means, it is generally true that most of the lesions resolve spontaneously.

If your child is bothered by the presence of this red mark, as could be expected, you should know several things about its treatment. First, try *not* to treat it! The naturally resolved strawberry mark is nearly invisible. However, almost anything done to these marks can leave a scar or permanent defect which later can look much worse than if it had been left alone. This is especially true for conventional surgical removal in which the marks look worse nearly every time. However, sometimes an early resolution can be initiated by a very light spray with liquid nitrogen, a freezing technique called *cryosurgery*.

In some children these strawberry lesions begin to grow rapidly after birth and can obstruct a vital organ such as the air passage in the throat or interfere with sight if they are near an eye. In these cases most dermatologists would choose to treat the child with large doses of cortisone to slow and reverse the growth of the spot. This method is not to be taken lightly, however, since cortisone has long-term side effects in some patients. It is advisable, therefore, to use this only with infants who have severe lesions.

DERMALERT

Strawberry marks will usually resolve slowly during childhood. The major problem associated with treating them is scarring; so surgical removal should be avoided if at all possible.

Q: We have an 8-month-old grandson with bright red spots on two of his fingers. The obstetrician said they would go away, but they appear to be spreading. Can they be removed, and at what age can something be done?

A: There are several angiomatous, or blood vessel-type, lesions which could occur in an 8-month-old. One of these is certainly the strawberry mark we have just mentioned. In that case strawberry marks have as good a chance of resolving on the fingers as they have on any other area. The key to treatment of your grandson's spots is the proper diagnosis. You must have him seen by a dermatologist to establish which type of blood vessel bumps these are; then the dermatologist may choose to treat them with cryosurgery or another method, or observe them if they are just strawberry angiomas. If they are getting larger, and he is only 8 months old, it would be wise to do that now because they will sometimes continue to get larger through infancy. But don't have them removed surgically, as I have said before, until they are evaluated by a dermatologist.

4

Skin Infections—Warts, Impetigo, and Other Common Skin Problems

Jane brought her 4-year-old in to me one day and said, "Looks like Troy has another selection from the 'Disease-of-the-Month' Club! Look at his rear."

I stood him up on the exam table (after an appropriate amount of hand holding and reassurance), pulled down his tiny Bermudas, and found little Troy's bottom literally covered with tiny dots of an infectious virus called *molluscum contagiosum*. Viral, bacterial, and yeast infections are the most common childhood diseases. Why? Because just as a child learns the ways of adults as he or she grows, the diminutive immune system is learning what is self and what is nonself, what is foreign and what is familiar. But in order to learn to protect the child's young body, each substance, infecting agent, or antigen must be experienced at least once. And that's why so many children get warts, molluscum, impetigo, diaper rashes, and a host of other infections. Most of these infections do heal without a trace, but you must know that some, such as impetigo, can have serious consequences if left untreated. We'll talk more about such consequences later in this chapter.

Molluscum

Q: What exactly are "molluscum spots"? How are they best treated?

A: Molluscum spots are caused by a large, brick-shaped virus that makes tiny one- to three-millimeter flesh-colored or pearly bumps grow on the skin. *Molluscum* means "soft body." That refers to the fact that these spots are not as hard and scaly as warts.

The second part of the name is "contagiosum," and you already have a sense for what *that* means. Anyone who touches this can grow his or her own set of molluscum lesions. They really like to grow in soft skin areas under armpits on children, but in adults they often occur in tender groin areas. Their propensity to strike the genital areas in adults has earned them the title of venereal disease, but that's really a misnomer, because most cases occur in children, and are therefore unrelated to sexual contacts.

DERMALERT

The pearly white bumps of molluscum contagiosum are very contagious and should be treated as soon as you find them. You can spot them by shining a flashlight tangential to the child's skin. This makes them show up very easily.

Many pediatricians question the need for treatment of molluscum contagiosum. They sometimes feel that, since they go away eventually, there's no need for vigorous therapy. But often, the child whose spots go untreated will spread the disease to his or her friends, just by simple hand-to-hand contact. So we usually treat them when we find them.

Treatment is directed at removing a small kernel of virus from the center of the bump, called the *molluscum body*. Once this is gone, the spots resolve without scarring. The molluscum body exudes virus out of the center of the lesion, and that's what causes them to spread. Results of one experiment suggested that these bumps resolved just by pricking them with a needle, but I've never been able to reproduce that success.

In the old days, dermatologists advised patients to sharpen a fingernail and flick off the bump, but this often resulted in infection. A successful modification of this was developed, however, in which the bump is frozen lightly with a cold spray and then scraped off with a tiny curved knife blade called a *curette*. This works, but will occasionally cause scarring.

In my experience, the most efficient removal requires cryosurgery (freezing) with liquid nitrogen. The nice part is that these spots don't need to be frozen as firmly as warts and therefore don't hurt quite so much. It's not necessary to scrape the lesions—an extremely light freeze is all that's needed. They really resolve beautifully with this treatment, without scarring.

Impetigo

Q: My daughter gets skin infections almost every summer. Our doctor says it's caused by strep bacteria. I thought these were what caused sore throat. Is there anything I can do to stop these?

A: Impetigo (often mistakenly called "infantigo") is an infection of the skin by dangerous strep or staph bacteria. These bacteria can indeed cause sore throats as well. Many children eventually have an episode or two of impetigo during the early years when young immune systems are developing.

Summertime is worst for impetigo. The heat makes moist skin fertile ground for the support of pathogenic (disease-producing) strains of bacteria. And exposed skin of children with infections enhances the spread of bacteria; that's why impetigo is thought to be so contagious.

Impetigo is a blistering disease. The spots start as reddish flat or bumpy spots which rapidly progress to blisters. The blisters break easily, weeping a clear, yellowish, infectious fluid which dries, forming the classic "honey-colored" crusts which tip off the dermatologist to the diagnosis.

While the infection of impetigo is seen as a local problem, some strep bacteria which cause it can also cause an inflammation of the kidneys known as *nephritis*. This risk is minimized through the use of oral antibiotics which must be taken for a full ten days for adequate protection.

Topical antibiotics also will help impetigo heal faster, but most dermatologists prescribe oral antibiotics to ensure that any pathogenic staph bacteria are completely wiped out, and to prevent nephritis developing from the strep bacteria.

DERMALERT

Impetigo bacteria can occasionally cause a severe kidney problem called nephritis. Treat it early, and for at least ten full days.

There are some general tips, though, which might help prevent impetigo. If your child seems susceptible, use an antibacterial soap for your family (though you should keep in mind that such soaps can be overly drying in winter).

Encourage your children to avoid contact with any children who have skin sores of any type. Contact with such sores causes impetigo. Tell your kids about the dangers of skin-to-skin contact with anyone who has sores.

If anyone in your family has frequent sore throats or nasal sores, ask your doctor to check them for pathogenic staph or strep; a family carrier could be seeding the disease among the children.

Make sure that any crusted sores on your children are examined early by a doctor. Treating one child early can prevent impetigo from developing in the others. If your child does contract impetigo, be sure to seek treatment before the child infects others.

Warts

Childhood warts are the bane of the dermatologist's existence. These nasty growths, called *verruca vulgaris*, are caused by the minuscule human papilloma virus.

The fact that they are caused by a virus means they are *contagious*. One of the most annoying problems in the office practice of dermatology is that pediatricians, family physicians, and other primary care doctors often advise that the lesions will fade on their own. While this may indeed be true in an isolated circumstance, read on before you decide to treat them with "watchful waiting."

A patient of mine I'll call Terry was entering the all-important third year of medical school when students get their first "hands-on" experience. But poor Terry couldn't conceive of it with *his* hands; we counted over 200 warts on his palms!

He told me a long and classic story about the development of warts. "When I was about 7 years old," he said, "I only had one wart on my wrist, but within the next few months, several new baby warts had developed around it. I was a real picker, Doc, and that seemed to spread them and make the warts multiply. I feel very embarrassed about examining patients with my hands like this, and I wondered what you could do."

Terry had waited too long. Now the job of removing his warts was a mammoth task instead of a minor inconvenience. The fact is that, while an isolated wart may indeed resolve, seemingly by magic (probably an immune or protective reaction by the body), others may develop from spread of the virus. That's the reason I try to lecture to pediatricians constantly about the natural history of warts. I encourage them to treat the warts or refer them for treatment earlier so that the final job is not such a colossal one. Ideally, I like to treat children before they can pick or chew at their warts and spread them around as Terry had done. I have actually seen children with *hundreds* of facial warts caused by biting finger warts!

DERMALERT

Picking and chewing at warts can spread these virus bumps all over one's face.

While an individual wart could be expected to go away on its own over a certain length of time (usually months to years), it is shedding virus constantly and possibly causing baby warts to develop which will also need to be treated. The key is, *don't wait*. Get your child to a dermatologist for treatment.

There is no magic age at which warts will resolve. If your

family practitioner or pediatrician cannot treat warts, then consult a dermatologist. Dermatologists can treat the problem in many different ways which we'll discuss later in this chapter.

You should know that the virus, although living in the warts, is technically *on* the body, it is not *in* the body or in the bloodstream.

DERMALERT

Beware of isolated warts. These warts are constantly shedding virus which can be spread elsewhere on your child and cause new warts. They should be treated as soon as you see them.

Q: I've heard it said many times that warts have roots and seeds. Don't you have to go into the wart to remove these?

A: This concept of warts growing like trees and plants is utter nonsense! The terminology got started long ago when scraped-off warts revealed a velvety rootlike surface below. Also, if you look down on a wart, you can see small dots in the surface of the wart which the old-timers called "seeds." But there are *no* seeds or roots in warts. The dots you see are merely thrombosed, or plugged, capillaries which feed the surface of the wart. Warts do not grow down into other tissues. In fact, each and every wart is a simple epidermal growth. That is, it grows in the most superficial layer of skin and never penetrates the dermis or second layer of skin. That's why they don't scar if they're removed carefully and gently.

Warts and Cancer

Q: The American Cancer Society always tells us to beware of any change in a wart or mole. Does that mean that warts can turn into skin cancer?

A: Common skin warts which we are apt to see on our children never turn into skin cancer. I repeat, common warts *never* turn into skin cancer! Two cases in which there is some suspicion that warts may be related to skin cancer both relate to genital warts, and we will talk more about those in Chapter 12.

Moles, however, are not infectious as are warts. They are cellular growths, often containing pigment. Moles rarely, but occasionally, do turn cancerous, and I'll discuss this more in Chapter 17. There you'll see a table comparing warts, moles, and melanomas, a type of skin cancer.

The real problem is that patients don't have the training to tell the difference between warts, moles, and skin cancers. That's why the American Cancer Society advises examination in any case where there's concern. The bottom line is that you probably don't have the expertise to tell the difference. Even dermatologists occasionally biopsy bumps which look strange and eventually turn out to be only warts. The "take-home" message is that you wouldn't want to assume that a skin cancer was a wart and not get it treated in time. When in doubt, call a skin expert!

Treatments for Warts

Q: What, then, can be done for these ugly warts?

A: There are about as many treatments for warts as there are patients who have them, and there is no one perfect treatment. The key words in wart therapy are "first do no harm," the physician's prime imperative. In short, when taking off warts, physicians don't want to cause a scar or mark that looks worse than the wart did or which lasts longer than the wart might have lasted. That's why we've largely abandoned treatments which burn off or cut off warts because of the scar left behind.

These days we rely on treatments which, although not uniformly successful the first time, can remove a wart dependably in most cases if the follow-up is adequate. Among these techniques is the application of various chemicals and/or acids to the wart surface in order to scale it off slowly. Many "wart removers" are available over the counter. They are much less effective than your doctor's treatments.

A 7-year-old boy named Jerry came in one day and his mother said that the large wart on his foot was finally going away under the influence of an over-the-counter substance. Since that was about the first time I had ever heard that a wart actually was making progress with this preparation, I was anxious to see the spot. When I pulled off Jerry's sock, I saw a large blistered heel wart with redness and tenderness almost up to his ankle! What had happened was immediately apparent. My one and only witnessed cure of this wart occurred because Jerry had gotten *allergic* to this medicine, not because it actually worked in its intended manner. This severe allergic reaction had blown the wart away (although quite painfully).

A popular way to remove warts is by the use of cryosurgery. This literally means "surgery with cold." In this technique, the skin is sprayed lightly with liquid nitrogen at the remarkable temperature of $-196°C$! Believe me, that's even colder than our average Lexington winter! This freezing method makes a small split or blister just below the wart. As the blister arises, the wart is pushed upward. Then the blister falls off, and if all parts of the wart were frozen adequately, the wart falls off with the blister top. Occasionally, with larger lesions, the technique has to be repeated several times at two- to three-week intervals.

But it's not all that easy with the freezing treatment. The freezing of small parts of the skin creates a miniature case of frostbite and that hurts! A year or two ago a little red-haired 6-year-old was trying to be a very brave soldier while I froze his huge finger warts. As I froze two or three of his larger warts, I could see tears forming, then I heard a plaintive little cry, and finally he looked up at me and growled, "You'd better stop it or I'm gonna call the police!"

Well, we froze the warts on that occasion and on one other and he did fine, without scars, but I'll never forget his warning. By the way, the police never came.

DERMALERT

Don't let anybody burn or cut off your child's warts. To do so is to risk scarring in almost every case. There are ways to remove these benign growths without permanently damaging the skin below.

Q: My 6-year-old daughter is plagued with warts. I have tried various preparations available, all with no results. She finally had to have them removed by freezing. This got rid of the ones she had at the time, but then they sprouted up in other areas. She's tried vitamin E topically to no avail. Is there some deficiency in her system that causes this, or what?

A: As a viral disease, warts can attack anyone who has skin, regardless of his or her diet. They recur sometimes because this virus may have already spread to other areas.

There is no magic vitamin or pill you can take to get rid of these warts. Rubbing them with vitamin E has no value whatsoever. The vitamin E therapy brings up a point, however: vitamin E seems to be the new folk remedy which has replaced some of the other old wives' tales used for years to treat warts.

Some of these are quite interesting. I have collected dozens of folk remedies for warts, including the following:

Rub the wart with a potato; then bury the potato in the backyard.

Ask your grandmother to buy your wart for a penny or a nickel (inflation has probably raised this to at least a quarter by now!).

Touch the warts with a dishrag; then bury the rag under the front steps.

Tie one knot in a string for each wart, and then drop the string over your shoulder by the light of a full moon.

Rub the wart with a piece of chalk (amazingly enough, this technique is actually practiced by more than one reputable dermatologist).

Paint stale stump water on the wart.

Rub the juice from a milkweed on the wart.

Have a hypnotist "exorcise" the wart.

All these techniques are accompanied by reports that on occasion they actually do work. This is the placebo effect in wart therapy: it is well known that, in rare instances, just the suggestion that a medicine will work actually brings on resolution of the lesion.

Obviously when the placebo effect works in warts, something has happened chemically to remove it, but as yet, no one knows what that something is. It may be a low-grade allergic reaction to the wart tissue itself.

What we really need is a wart vaccine. However, this tiny virus cannot yet be cultured or grown outside the human body, so this is, as yet, not possible. Work proceeds in this direction, however. Some investigators have derived a vaccine by grinding up wart tissue and administering it by injection, but other researchers warn that this may be a very dangerous practice. You see, the wart virus is a DNA virus, and DNA is that stuff that controls all cell mechanisms. No one wants extra DNA in his or her system since it might be possible that it could cause cancers and/or other problems.

DERMALERT

Don't get a wart vaccine, even if you're offered one. They're far from safe, probably don't work, and may even cause other problems. The future may hold promise in this direction, but only after much more research is done.

Fingernail Warts

Q: I have a wart growth on both sides of my little finger, and it is now growing under the nails. I use a cuticle clipper occasionally to get rid of the hardness on either side of the nail. What do you suggest?

A: First of all, give up your cuticle clipper. Cutting into these warts may cause localized infection. You also get wart virus on the clippers and may spread warts around if you use them in other areas. And worse yet, anyone who uses your clippers can get them. I've seen them spread like wildfire through whole families by this very route. The difficulty with warts around the nails (periungual warts) is that the virus hides under the free edge of the nail and is almost impossible to get rid of by freezing in this location. Often, freezing is used to reduce the size of the warts so that other therapies can be used.

For periungual warts (the most difficult to treat anywhere), I have found very little which is completely effective. One of the best agents used for this process is DNCB (dinitrochlorobenzene). this compound is a type of topically, or surface-applied medicine which is highly allergenic. That is, the body very easily forms an allergic reaction to it in much the same way it reacts to poison ivy. The medicine is applied in very dilute form to a "sensitization area," such as the inside of the wrist, once a day until that area reacts and itches. Then the treatment period starts. A small amount of DNCB is rubbed onto the warts and is poked in gently with a wooden toothpick. This activates an allergic reaction in and around the wart, and intense inflammation in the area apparently wipes out the wart.

Recently, two new sensitizers have been used to treat warts by this same principle. These are poison ivy resin and squaric acid dibutylester. You should ask your dermatologist about the use of these agents and the possibility for curing your warts. It may take several months, including multiple applications, to cause the allergy, but after it occurs, treatment of the warts is a simple process of applying the medicine repeatedly. Naturally, the poison ivy resin therapy is *never* to be used by anyone who is not *already* allergic to the stuff. Since contact with poison ivy could occur in the future, dermatologists don't want to sensitize patients to it when other treatments will do.

Plantar (Sole) Warts

Q: For twenty-nine years, I have had a plantar wart on each foot. I have had every treatment for them from x-rays to cauterization, but I was advised against surgery because I have been told that scar tissue can be as painful, if not more so, than the wart.

The situation got so bad that I could hardly put my feet on the floor in the morning, so I saw a surgeon who suggested shoes that were sculptured to my feet. I have worn these shoes for fourteen years and have had relative comfort. However, I can never go barefoot for fear of infecting my family. I still curl my toes under to relieve the pressure and actually turn my feet over to the outside so that I do not walk on them.

A: Some dermatologists say that they would rather see a minor case of skin cancer than a plantar wart. Plantar warts are ordinary skin warts which have grown on the sole. The term "plantar" simply refers to the plantar, or bottom, surface of the foot as opposed to the volar, or top surface. It has nothing to do with the word "planter." These warts are tough to get rid of because they are pushed into the skin rather than being allowed to grow out above the foot. They do *not* have roots which grow into or around bones, or penetrate the actual foot substance. They are *surface* growths which are just pushed inward. But since they are located in a weight-bearing area, they can be very painful and are difficult to treat.

Cryosurgery cannot be used on the foot in most instances because it's too painful and much less effective in this particular location. While x-ray therapy often does work in up to 85 percent of single warts, treatment is reserved only for the most recalcitrant or stubborn single warts.

Obviously, one worries about the long-term effects of radiation on the bones and inner tissues of the foot, such as cancer, ulcers, and scarring. But a recent study in the dermatologic literature of some 7,000 patients showed x-ray treatment to be extremely safe therapy. However, most dermatologists have given up this treatment because having an x-ray unit in their offices hugely increases their liability insurance.

Let me warn you very strongly against having surgery on the bottom of the foot. This almost always causes a permanent scar which can actually hurt more than the original wart, because of pressure exerted upon it while walking.

So we turn to other therapies for these stubborn warts on the soles. Among the old-fashioned but effective remedies for plantar warts is a substance called *podophyllin*. Podophyllin is a plant resin which kills the rapidly multiplying skin cells which contain the wart virus. Its irritating action works on plantar warts only when it is bandaged onto the wart for extended times (sometimes ten to fourteen days). Used in this way, it can effectively eliminate a wart if the pain is not too disagreeable. Be very careful to ask your doctor how much pain might be involved. If you need to step on the brake of your car firmly, you could have an accident if the pain prevents you from doing so, or it could interfere with your job if you must spend a lot of time on your feet.

After the initial podophyllin treatment, which removes the body of the wart, I use a technique that we call "F&S" therapy, which stands for "formalin and salicylic acid." This is one of the few techniques which is successful in removing large, multiple, or mosaic plantar warts. It involves painting the wart each night with a solution of formaldehyde. The wart is then covered with a plaster of salicylic acid, which helps the medicine penetrate into the wart. This is repeated every night, and over a few weeks the wart dries out thoroughly and starts to scale. Sometimes the drying is severe enough to cause splits in the skin; this can be painful temporarily. In this case, the medicine is stopped for a few days, then resumed.

During this treatment your dermatologist will see you every few weeks to pare down the superficial dead skin and check to see if there is any residual wart. You will then be told if you need to continue the treatment.

The F&S technique has defeated the largest wart I have ever seen, a huge three-by-five-inch wart which covered nearly the entire sole! The patient, Judy, who had this huge wart had been treated with every known therapy, including cryosurgery, the pain of which I decided to risk because of the disability caused by this monster wart. She couldn't walk anyway, so in this case the blisters could not be any more painful. Since she had had to put up with this wart since she had been a toddler, she was willing to try anything. That's when I decided to try the formalin therapy suggested by a dermatologist friend from Tallahassee.

DERMALERT

Formalin is poisonous if taken internally. Do not make any attempt to smell this medicine because it is quite irritating to the nasal passages. Take special precautions to keep this and all medicines out of the reach of your children. You can use it on your children safely, but don't let the bottle get into their hands. This technique should only be used when supervised by a dermatologist skilled in its use.

After she was put on the formalin therapy, Judy disappeared from my office until approximately a year later. When she came back for me to check another skin problem, I asked her if I could take a look at her wart. She grinned coyly and took off her shoe. I was flabbergasted. The only trace that there had ever been a wart in the area was a small scar where she had attempted to have the wart cut off years before I treated her. She said that her wart resolved slowly over several months of using this special F&S therapy. We were both thrilled and amazed at this incredible result.

Q: How do people get warts on their feet? Does going barefoot have anything to do with it?

A: I want to stress that warts occur on the bottom of the feet only because people *do* go barefoot. In fact, that may be the *only* way people catch them. Therefore, even at home, and certainly in public places like swimming pools, hotels, and gymnasium locker rooms, *do not go barefoot*. The best protection against contracting warts in pool areas or gyms is to wear rubber thongs, or "flip-flops." They can stop the skin from picking up this nuisance virus.

Frustrating Facial Warts

Q: My son has "flat warts" on his face. Is there a way to treat these without freezing them?

A: Yes. Recently there have been good reports on 5-fluorouracil (5-FU) cream, a medicine used in the elderly to remove premalignant sunspots. It is also reliable for removing flat warts on the face. It does this by slowing the multiplication of the wart-containing cells and by inducing irritation in the warts themselves. This cream, while slightly irritating to the skin, does a fine job in many instances. Ask your doctor about it. When using this medicine, stay out of the sun. This drug is made more potent and irritating by the sun's rays. If you get an irritation instead of a cure from it, call your doctor.

DERMALERT

Facial warts should be treated as soon as possible because they spread rapidly. Ask your dermatologist to tell you about Efudex (5-FU) cream for their treatment.

5

##

Eczema—How to Put Out the Fire on Your Child's Skin

Although it's possible to write an entire book on the subject of childhood eczema, I'll attempt to give you the salient features of the disease and the treatments which can help.

Common eczema of childhood is usually called *atopic eczema*. Atopic means "altered reactivity." This means that affected children have a family tendency to develop dry, itchy skin which scales and cracks. Often it forms large infected patches on the fronts of the elbows and the backs of the knees.

To illustrate how severe the problem can be, I would like to tell you about a 5-year-old named Andy who was brought to me when I was a resident at the Medical College of Georgia. When I entered the room, all I could see was the blur of Andy's hands scratching his skin almost everywhere. Hardly a square inch of his body was spared from the torture of atopic eczema. Some areas were so bad that they were split open widely and literally dripping pus from scratch marks he had made. Andy's mother was in a real tizzy, scolding him almost constantly to stop scratching. She did not know that he was literally unable to stop scratching when his skin was that inflamed.

37

I questioned his mother about his problem, and it seems that he had had trouble with itchy skin ever since infancy. At that time he had what they thought was a severe case of cradle cap which never cleared up. With time it had spread severely to the fronts of the arms, the backs of the knees, and the neck area. Most recently, during the Georgia summer heat, it had become infected, compounding the problem.

She told me that Andy's father had had asthma and hay fever and that most of the family had severe sinus troubles. These are common associated findings in the families of children with atopic eczema.

Further questioning revealed some reasons why Andy's eczema failed to clear up under the care of his pediatrician. His mother said that when Andy was an infant, the pediatrician had recommended a potent antibacterial soap. His mother thought that since this was recommended by his pediatrician it was a good *treatment* for atopic eczema. Actually, the soap had only irritated it. She had also been bathing him three times a day! No wonder the little tyke had skin as dry and cracked as the Mojave Desert! She had been washing out all of his natural skin oils for *years*.

DERMALERT

Children with dry scaly eczema should have *fewer* baths, not more! Irritating antibacterial soaps should be completely eliminated. A *superfatted* soap should be used.

I began a three-pronged attack to save poor Andy's skin. First, since all his scratch marks were badly infected, an internal antibiotic was absolutely required.

Second, since his main problem was skin dryness, I cut him down to one bath per week and changed him to Dove soap (other superfatted soaps are fair too) if he used any soap at all. Baby soap is okay, too, in moderation; but I see problems due to overuse of it in cases where it's assumed to be harmless. Some kids do even better by avoiding soap altogether and rubbing on a little Cetaphil lotion until a lather almost forms, then wiping it off with a tissue or towel, leaving most of this wonderful moisturizing lotion right on the skin.

Let me digress a minute to tell you a little story about a child who was treated by the renowned dermatologist Dr. J. Lamar Callaway at Duke University. One day he prescribed a "generic" cream for a child with eczema as bad as Andy's. The cream was in a large one-pound jar which he dispensed for a few cents to the family along with instructions to apply it thinly to all eczema areas twice daily.

The child returned two weeks later with almost complete healing of his eczema, and Mom demanded, "What was in that 'mystery cream' of yours?"

"Just a little stuff we call 'Cream V' around here, that's all," he said.

"Cream V?" she asked, "What's the V stand for? I want to know what I'm putting on my child!"

"Well, if you must know," he said, "the V stands for plain, pure vegetable shortening, right off the supermarket shelf!"

It's true! It works! It's probably one of the best and safest moisturizers ever found, although not very aesthetically acceptable. But Dr. Callaway had found, over the years, that mothers just wouldn't use the stuff if they knew it was vegetable shortening, no matter how effective it was. That's why he started calling it Cream V.

Third, getting back to Andy, I started him on a hydrocortisone cream just strong enough to cool the fires of inflammation burning in his eczema.

These principles are very important in the treatment of your child. The fact is that Andy probably had atopic eczema because he had the wrong ancestors. The disease definitely is hereditary. We know that children of families having a lot of sinus trouble, allergies, hay fever, rhinitis, and hives have a greater incidence, or frequency, of atopic eczema.

The fact that eczema victims may have allergies of other types does not mean that an allergy causes the eczema. This skin disease seems to be completely independent of allergies that are usually treated with shots and desensitization. In atopic dermatitis these methods are of very little use.

The primary fact to be remembered in atopic dermatitis is that these kids itch, and so they *will* scratch! There is absolutely no use whatsoever in telling a child with this problem not to scratch these spots. The disease itches so intensely that the child has little or no choice whether or not to react to the itching. They actually scratch hard enough to scrape open the skin because the pain induced by scratching and tearing away at the skin is actually *more tolerable* than the itch itself!

DERMALERT

Itching is one of the most intolerable forms of misery. We scratch to injure the skin because that pain is more tolerable than the itching!

Treating the Itch of Eczema

One of my dermatology professors used to say that the itching of eczema was one of the most disagreeable sensations a human being could have. He had a neat trick for solving the scratching dilemma. After prescribing a medicated cream for patients (to cut down on inflammation), he advised them to put a little of the cream on the flat of the finger pad and to actually rub it into the itchy spot as many times a day as was needed. In this way he allowed the patients to do a "modified scratch" without injuring the skin. He also got the remarkable bonus of applying the topical cortisone cream in a very efficient manner, that is, rubbed well into the skin. This technique has worked so well for me during my years in practice that I use it for virtually every patient with an itching problem.

DERMALERT

Do you have an itchy skin rash? You may be able to solve it by rubbing in your *medicine* with the flat of the finger pads. *But don't use your nails!* You'll badly damage the skin.

It's not hard to see from the description of the itch involved in eczema that it does no good whatsoever to admonish or scold a child for scratching. This only increases the guilt of the child and the guilt of the parents, who usually mistakenly assume that they have somehow given their child this disease through something they have done. Eczema is an unfortunate problem of children (and of some adults), and it would be unwise to punish our children or ourselves because of their misfortune in contracting this terrible disease.

Although some children do grow out of childhood eczema, the problem often evolves into a chronic smoldering eczema of the neck or hands as the patient ages. While cortisone creams can help the inflammation, it is often necessary, as I've suggested, to prescribe antibiotics because of the infection that occurs in eczema scratch marks. Don't worry too much if your doctor keeps your child on antibiotics for a significant length of time: very few cases of severe eczema will clear without them. Topical antibiotics can occasionally be of help, but you run some risk of sensitizing your child or making him or her allergic to the neomycin and other ingredients in these drugs. So if your doctor gives your child a topical antibiotic and if a worse rash develops instead of steadily clearing, the doctor should consider a possible allergic reaction to the topical antibiotic. I use topical antibiotics for my patients, but very selectively.

DERMALERT

Topical antibiotics don't work as well as oral ones. Occasionally, the ingredients in topicals can cause severe skin allergies.

Finally, you asked about the effect of sun on eczema. Sun, in general, does not help. A child with eczema needs moisture and general skin care to improve. The real reason why kids with eczema do better during the seasons of the year when the sun is brightest (spring and summer) is because of the increased *humidity*, not the sunlight. These children do not need the damaging rays of the sun.

6

Poison Ivy—
Leave These Leaves Alone!

"Leaves of three, leave it be!" Everyone's heard that old adage, but unfortunately, not enough of us heed its wise advice. There are few more uncomfortable patients than those with a severe case of poison ivy.

If you doubt how prevalent this affliction is, just look at the full shelf of over-the-counter remedies for it in the drugstore. It seems as if a new remedy springs up each year. Poison ivy is a problem, certainly, but one that can be prevented and treated very effectively if it does occur.

Poison ivy is a form of allergic contact dermatitis. This means that the skin gets allergic to the thick oily resin of the poison ivy plant. In order to do this, the resin from the broken leaf of the plant must streak across the skin. The resin can also be picked up by vectors such as tools, clothing, shoes, dogs, cats, golf clubs, and so forth which have touched the resin and have not been cleaned thoroughly afterward.

Scientists have found substances similar to poison ivy resin in Egyptian mummy tombs, and even after 3,000 years, the substance can still cause dermatitis! But it's really not hard to get rid of. Since the substance which causes the allergy is a thick oily resin, soapy water washes it away completely. No special soap is needed. Some people foolishly resort to using chlorine bleach, turpentine, and gasoline for removing poison ivy. This is completely unnecessary and can be quite irritating to the skin.

DERMALERT

Plain soap and water are all that are needed to remove the dangerous poison ivy resin from skin or household items.

Q: Can we get the disease from touching the blister fluid that comes out of the spots of poison ivy?

A: Absolutely not. There is no way that the blister fluid from poison ivy can cause disease in another person or, in fact, even spread it on the victim, if the lesions have been washed with soap and water since initial contact with the resin.

Of course, this probably was not true in the old days when that theory got started. In those days, people only washed about once a week. After several days, when their blisters began to weep, they still had the sticky resin which had not been washed off. So they indeed got new spots of poison ivy from the blister fluid, but this was purely by accident.

Remember: Be sure to wash off any item—animal, child, tool, or anything else—that has come in contact with the poison ivy resin, and you'll get fewer and fewer lesions instead of spreading the spots.

DERMALERT

A ten-minute rule for poison ivy, after exposure to the weed: if you wash the area well, rinsing within ten minutes, you may not even get the disease.

Q: I was on a picnic where I knew I got into poison ivy but it didn't break out for two days after this. Can you explain this fact?

A: Since poison ivy is a disease of the immune system, it takes a finite length of time, usually two days or so, if a patient has had the disease before, to erupt on the skin in the classic streaked, red, itchy blisters. For this reason, dermatologists often call poison ivy the "Tuesday disease," because most cases show up in our offices on a Tuesday or Wednesday following picnics or outings on weekends.

There are even some dermatologists who refer to poison ivy as "the widow's weed." Widows often go out to their husbands' gravesites on Sunday afternoons to tend the grass and overgrowth around the grave. Here they often come in contact with poison ivy. Always be careful in clearing underbrush, since poison ivy often thrives in these areas.

Unnoticed exposure to poison ivy has been recognized by dermatologists for many years. Dr. Alexander Fisher, a renowned contact dermatitis specialist, is quite adept at tracing down contact exposure to weird substances, including various plants. He once had an elderly woman patient with an extremely tough case of apparent skin allergy. He suspected poison ivy but could not find the source. Finally, at lunchtime one day, Dr. Fisher went out to the patient's house and searched for sources of contact exposure. Every room in the house proved clean as a whistle. As he was leaving, the lady asked him if he would come see her beautiful growth of English ivy which she had cultivated for many years. As they rounded the corner of the house, Dr. Fisher gasped at what he saw. Her "English ivy" was a pure, undiluted culture of poison ivy plants. She had very carefully cultivated her "ivy" over the years, trimming, watering daily, and fertilizing it. After each exposure she developed more dermatitis. She apparently never realized it was due to her English ivy because of the delay between exposure and development of the rash.

DERMALERT

Poison ivy takes about two days to show up on the skin; so any rash that appears is related to something you touched two or more days ago.

Q: I don't catch poison ivy, even if I handle the stuff. But recently someone told me that I could still get the disease. Is he right?

A: He certainly is. There are people who are known to develop poison ivy dermatitis even after years of thinking they cannot get it. The immune system is pretty smart. It learns how to recognize a substance as a foreign, allergy-causing agent. That culmination of the training of the immune system can occur at any time, even after years of intermittent exposure.

Q: I always put calamine lotion on my kids' poison ivy, but it seems to take so long to work. I have tried the cortisone creams I can buy in the drugstore, but they don't seem to do much either. What's best?

A: Avoidance is the best way to treat poison ivy. Admittedly, this is hard to do because of the varying look of the plants from time to time. Sometimes it grows as a shiny, three-leafed vine, and sometimes it stands alone like a tiny shrub.

Calamine is the age-old remedy for poison ivy. It does dry the lesions slightly and sometimes calms itching. But most of us feel that it really just covers up the sores so they're not so apparent. Personally, I think it's not worth the mess. As a matter of fact, no one has ever improved upon tap water soaks to help speed along healing of the blistering stage of poison ivy. Note that I said *tap* water. It doesn't help a bit to add anything to it (although some southern dermatologists recommend adding a small amount of bourbon to the tap water and then drinking it!). But clear water compresses without soap do help the acute stage.

Using topical hydrocortisone on poison ivy lesions functions more to mask the diagnostic signs of the disease than it does to help the itchy rash. In fact, the amount of hydrocortisone in the available over-the-counter cream is much too low to help the severe dermatitis of poison ivy. However, it can modify its appearance so that when you do see a dermatologist, an exact diagnosis may not be possible, since the skin rash can then look more like hives than poison ivy. In some cases it is almost impossible to tell the difference, except by watching the untreated lesions over a few days. When they blister, the correct diagnosis becomes obvious.

DERMALERT

If you have any irritation of the skin, don't apply anything to it until you see your dermatologist. You may mask the signs needed to make the diagnosis correctly.

You should also know that using topical antihistamines and numbing agents such as those ending in "-caine" or "-dryl" can result in worsening of your dermatitis if you get allergic to various substances in these medications. This includes vitamin E, which can cause severe dermatitis if an allergic reaction develops because of its use.

Q: I got poison ivy in the winter once. How could that be?

A: Amazingly, many patients get poison ivy from their firewood. They think, mistakenly, that the logs are entangled by simple vines, but these vines are often poison ivy branches. Remember, the stems of the poison ivy plant still contain active resin even in the coldest of winters! That means if you carry in branches of poison ivy with your logs, you can look like a red blistered balloon a couple of days later.

DERMALERT

Resin-contaminated firewood is the most common cause of winter poison ivy.

Q: I find that most of the over-the-counter remedies work quite well within two weeks to heal my attacks of poison ivy. Why not just use drugstore items to treat it?

A: Your question is a classic example of a mistaken "cause-and-effect" relationship. While many products available without a prescription may seem to help, these agents probably do nothing to improve upon the rate of healing of the poison ivy. If you would just let your case of poison ivy go untreated for a while, you would then see that the poison ivy rash decreases dramatically in almost every case within two weeks.

7

—

The War Against Acne—
A Struggle to
Save Face

Every month I see hundreds of teenagers who are battling their way through a desperate fight which, for some, will last for all their teen years and even beyond. That fight occurs as nature starts to create for them supple, adult skin lubricated and ready for the rest of their lives.

I've always felt it a shame that most people fail to realize how important a teen's face is to him or her. Day after day I see kids who won't talk, won't socialize, won't even look at me sometimes, because they're so ashamed of their appearance.

In fact, I'm sure that acne is one reason why I'm so dedicated to dermatology. As faces clear, I often see personalities blossom on subsequent office visits just like time-lapse pictures of an opening rose. What a delightful experience for a physician to see children climb out of the sadness that is acne.

The real problem with acne is delay—delay in talking over the situation with parents, and delay in seeking *dermatologic* help. Early help from a dermatologist for severe acne can save not only a youngster's skin but the psyche as well.

Q: My 16-year-old daughter has been seeing a dermatologist for the past two years. She's used a variety of medicines, both topically and internally. These include antibiotics (tetracycline), benzoyl peroxide, and Retin-A. We don't see much improvement. Is this unusual? She is very, very discouraged.

A: Acne is a disease which can last for years in some teens. It's a process in which the tiny tubes leading from the oil glands become completely or partially plugged. This results in back pressure on the oil glands themselves and trapping of bacteria. These bacteria are called *Propionibacterium acnes*. These *P. acnes* bacteria do not actually cause an infection, but the bacteria multiply within the oil gland, producing an enzyme called *lipase* which splits oil into very irritating substances called *fatty acids*. These cause irritation of the oil gland lining and eventual rupture of the oil gland, resulting in what appears as a red acne bump.

DERMALERT

Acne is *not* an infection. The few bacteria present in acne bumps really just help break down oil in the oil gland.

Treatments

There are thousands of treatments for teenage complexion problems. Choosing the right ones from among the many over-the-counter and prescription products is the most important therapeutic dilemma in acne treatment. Let's look at a few types.

Antibiotics

There are reasons why your dermatologist has used each of the substances in your daughter's treatment. First of all, tetracycline is good and it has been used in acne therapy for years. It has two functions. The first of these is to kill off the *P. acnes* bacteria. Happily, they are exquisitely sensitive to that medicine. Also, the tetracycline appears to be an inhibitor of the enzyme lipase, which causes rotting of the oil below the surface. In short, it's a bump stopper.

Benzoyl Peroxide

Topical benzoyl peroxide has several uses in acne. Some consider its main function one of a drying and peeling agent, but it appears now that it's a much more remarkable substance than we had first realized. Besides drying out acne, it actually inhibits the growth of *P. acnes* bacteria. There are many forms of benzoyl peroxide, of course. The best are the acetone and water gel formulations and some can be bought over the counter.

Retin-A

Retin-A cream is a form of vitamin A acid applied topically. It appears to correct the defect in the oil gland lining which causes plugging of the canal. However, Retin-A can be an irritating substance. I've had some patients complain of redness when they were on it. But many dermatologists, including myself, prescribe Retin-A, especially in whitehead and blackhead acne. If you *can* tolerate it, it will do the job.

Some concern has recently arisen about the advisability of using Retin-A; this was prompted by a study showing that Retin-A could cause skin cancers in the presence of sunlight. This study was carried out using a very concentrated solution of Retin-A on rats chosen for their special sun sensitivity. Other studies have shown that Retin-A may *protect* one from skin cancers, so any resolution is far from final. However, there is now a published warning concerning the use of Retin-A in acne patients who are exposed to a lot of sun. Since Retin-A does cause some thinning of the dead protective layer of the skin, patients are advised not to use it when they are going to be in the sunlight for extended periods.

Attitude and Acne

If your child's acne doesn't improve with treatment, the answer may lie in three different areas. First, he or she may not be performing all the treatments required by the dermatologist. Take my patient Ronnie, for instance, who was literally dragged into my office by his mother. She pushed him into the corner and said, "Treat his acne!" Ronnie was a surly young high school student who was covered with "zits." He really needed help, but I could see he was not about to accept it. I tried to treat him by giving him a lotion which required him to do very little, but this approach failed. Ronnie was certain that the world owed him a smooth, pimple-free face, and that he should not have to work for it.

His mother persisted, and month after month he was brought back for reexamination, but he continued to have more and more severe nodular acne and began to scar in spite of my care.

Then one day Ronnie took a complete turnabout and came in by himself to talk to me. He had found a girl for whom he'd developed a romantic interest, but was afraid she wouldn't like him if he had a crater face. Now he wanted help.

The change was remarkable. Over the next few months Ronnie began using his topical treatments and taking his capsules, and he continued to improve, with very few permanent scars. After one year, he was well stabilized, and his skin looked beautiful. I then began decreasing his medications until he was discharged. Today he's in college with a clear face. I still see him from time to time to treat other minor skin problems, and he never fails to thank me.

DERMALERT

> It's highly unlikely that your dermatologist can clear your or your child's acne unless the patient is willing to expend the effort required to *get* clear.

Q: I sometimes wonder if my daughter's acne is not clearing up because she doesn't like her doctor.

A: Motivation is needed on both sides of the treatment program. In short, the rapport between the physician and patient is more important in acne than it is in almost any other skin disease. The disease moves rapidly in many patients, leaving its tracks for all to see. It's absolutely crucial that a child have a good working relationship with the dermatologist. If not, it's time to move on to another dermatologist.

Dr. Marsh, my mentor in dermatology, once told me, "Joe, if

you can't learn to love treating acne, don't ever get into dermatology. Clearing a kid's acne is a real thrill for me. It'll do the same for you if you learn to treat it and love treating it!" He was right.

The bottom line concerning your daughter's case is that if you feel uncomfortable for any reason with the treatment or the rate at which her condition improves, you should discuss it with the dermatologist. This can only help to clarify any questions.

Diet and Acne

Q: What can I do to get my pimples to go away? Is it my diet?

A: Diet is of much less importance than we used to think in acne care. The majority of dermatologists today recommend a well balanced diet but no definite dietary restrictions. Many of us, however, myself included, recommend avoidance of dairy products, including milk, cheese, and ice cream, and pork, including bacon and sausage. There must be an agent in these products which encourages acne to form, because patients do better when they avoid them. But as far as I'm concerned, my patients can have all the chocolate, Cokes, candy, nuts, Fritos, potato chips, french fries, and hamburgers that they want.

Research shows that there is no significant change in acne caused by eating chocolate. In fact, several years ago, a major study was done by Dr. Albert M. Kligman, a well respected dermatologist and researcher. The study, published in the December 15, 1969, *Journal of the American Medical Association,* was performed at the University Hospital in Philadelphia, Pennsylvania.

Dr. Kligman gave 1,200 calories of chocolate each day to one group of sixty-five acne-prone patients and 1,200 calories per day of nonchocolate-containing lookalike and taste-alike bars to a matched group. No one, not even the researcher, knew which kids were getting the real or fake chocolate. All the kids were watched for new acne bumps.

After many weeks, the researchers discovered that there was *no* significant difference between the two groups. So it's true; chocolate's *not* the acne answer.

However, in my own practice, if patients complain that every time they eat a chocolate bar they get new bumps, I tell them quite frankly that they would be fools to continue eating *anything* they think causes new lesions.

You see, on a microscopic level, it takes over two to three weeks to make an acne bump; so it's impossible to get all those changes overnight after eating a suspected acne inducer. Maybe someday we'll find out that foods may trigger acne, but in order to do so, we'll have to work with a three-week (or more) history of what was eaten. And that's so difficult that the long-term studies have never been done, except for chocolate.

DERMALERT

Chocolate does not affect acne.

Soaps

Q: I've been using a glycerine soap for my acne. Is that best for oily acne skin?

A: Regular glycerine soap is really quite mild. In many of my cases of severe acne, it's much *too* mild. And for some people it's been found to be frankly comedogenic (whitehead-causing). For my patients, I like mild drying soaps containing sulfur or benzoyl peroxide. I think a mild general drying soap tends to dehydrate the oil gland opening, temporarily enlarging it, allowing normal passage of oil to occur. That's why many of the medications that dermatologists recommend do cause surface drying. One popular manufacturer does make a glycerine *acne* soap, but I still prefer the mild drying soaps.

Emotions—Can They "Scare" Up Acne?

Q: Can stress provoke acne? I had a disturbing breakup with my boyfriend and my acne got much worse.

A: As a *general rule,* I would say that emotions do not have much to do with acne development. The disease is one of plugged oil glands and no one has yet determined how emotional factors could have a relationship there.

However, in *practice,* I find that acne often worsens around exam times and other times of severe stress. We are still not sure if this results from the actual stress having a physiological effect on the acne, or whether a person just thinks about the acne more during stressful times, possibly pressing or picking at the bumps with greater frequency, or generally ignoring total skin care because of the stress.

DERMALERT

As a rule, stress has very little to do with skin conditions. However, acne and a few other conditions often worsen in times of emotional stress and tension.

Healing Time

Q: Why is it that I've been on my acne treatment program of tetracycline and applied lotions and medicines for two weeks and I haven't seen much change? Why am I still getting a few new bumps?

A: In these days of air travel, almost everyone has heard of the time delay, called *jet lag,* in which the body does not adjust quickly enough as one moves from time zone to time zone. The same thing can happen in acne therapy. Some of us have dubbed this time delay between the onset of treatment and the onset of improvement as "zit lag." It's during this period that the skin is adapting to the medicines your dermatologist has prescribed; it can take some two to six weeks before you begin to show an improvement. This is especially true with such agents as topical vitamin A acid and topical antibiotics which have a built-in waiting period before their therapeutic action begins. If you're still not improving nicely four to six weeks down the road, discuss modifications or changes in your acne treatment program with your doctor.

DERMALERT

Acne medications do not work instantaneously. Allow a period of some weeks for your body to adjust to the medications and start healing.

Acne in Older Persons

Q: I'm a 40-year-old male with hard lumps and bumps on my face which appear from time to time. Most of the time these are near the nose. These spots seem to begin as pimples but never surface. Often after a couple of weeks they are no longer sore.

If these bumps are not aggravated by mashing or sticking with a needle, they stay under the skin! What should I do?

A: These lumps are acne. Acne is not a disease of teenagers only. We're seeing more and more cases of acne (even the more severe nodulocystic kind that you appear to have) in people well beyond their teenage years. Although we think a lot of this has to do with the use of cosmetics by women, we suspect that acne persists in men because of the constant presence of large amounts of male hormone.

One thing about your question is quite disturbing. You should *never* operate on your own cysts! Squeezing, mashing, or needling these cysts can not only cause a severe infection (when infection may not have been present originally), but it can increase scarring by injecting the rotting cyst material into the surrounding skin.

And, needless to say, using a needle on your cysts is to be avoided at all costs. Metal objects can transmit severe infections and even hepatitis. Never approach your face with the intention of doing your own "acne surgery."

DERMALERT

If an acne bump is squeezed, often 10 percent of the rotting material in the bump is ejected onto the surface and 80 to 90 percent is injected into the skin below, causing a worsening inflammation and possible scarring. The "two thumbs" technique is the *worst* way to treat an acne bump.

Acne Induced by Physical Pressure

Q: My husband has had acne on his back for a long time. He is now 30 years old, and I would like to know if it will ever go away.

A: Acne can be a process which does not resolve until middle age in some men. While there are not very many 65-year-olds with acne, it's impossible to tell the individual patient when his or her own case of acne will subside. We believe that treatment of acne may keep the patient asymptomatic; that is, the patient may have a tendency for the condition to occur, but this tendency is effectively masked while the disease essentially burns itself out. Treatment, in other words, is a protective screen in front of the acne forest fire, and we keep the screen up as long as necessary to prevent damage. Although I cannot tell your husband when he will lose his acne, I can tell him that almost everyone does indeed stop forming new bumps as they age.

More to the point, you should look for the causes of your husband's back acne. I treated a salesman with back acne who had no lesions whatsoever on his face. But he drove about 500 to 800 miles a week, and he thought that might have something to do with the extensive acne on his back.

Sure enough, when we went out to examine his car, we found it had vinyl seat covers. He found that after sitting on this occlusive surface for some time, his back was very hot and sweaty. When I started him on a treatment regimen, I also advised him to get a soft sheepskin cover for his seat. This resulted in a very prompt resolution of his back acne.

The most striking case I have ever seen of pressure-induced acne was in a young woman named Sherry who had very severe acne on the right cheek only. The bumps were so close together that her whole cheek was covered with papular, or small bump, acne.

I asked her if she leaned her face on her hand. Sherry said she was very careful not to do this because she thought that might have something to do with her condition.

I put Sherry on a treatment program but she didn't do very well. The explosive acne continued to develop in exactly the same area. One day her husband came in with her when I was asking her about local influences on the skin.

I asked her again if something was pressing on the skin of the right side of her face. Her husband then blurted out the fact that she slept on her right hand every single night.

Now it was clear that Sherry's hand was causing her acne. So I prescribed a soft, brown garden glove for her to wear only at night and asked her to try to keep her pillow between her hand and her face. Sherry's acne cleared almost magically. Since then I've been quite impressed with the effect of pressure on the skin in causing acne.

DERMALERT

Anything which presses on or heats up the skin can cause a more severe eruption. This applies not only to vinyl seat backs, but to anything which occludes the skin, such as leaning on your hand.

Q: My son is on the football team and he's getting acne much worse than last year on his forehead and chin areas. Is there an explanation?

A: The problem your son is having may be helmet and chin-strap acne. Sometimes it is extraordinarily difficult to get these areas cleared without stopping the pressure by the strap. Drying agents used on the forehead and chin during football season can help calm the eruption, but for the most part, it's necessary to alleviate the pressure. This can be done by padding the chin-strap area and helmet contact points with a very soft felt material. It's not perfect, but it may help.

Dermatopathic Lymphadenopathy

Q: I have a lot of bumps on my chin and mouth area. Some of these go under my chin onto my neck and the glands in my neck are enlarged. Why would this be?

A: This condition is called *dermatopathic lymphadenopathy*. This means that the tiny lymph glands under the chin area are draining the products of inflammation from your acne areas. These products lodge temporarily within the glands and cause them to swell. The lumps can get quite tender and sometimes persist until the acne itself has come under control. The presence of inflammation in the lymph glands of the neck will often lead your dermatologist to consider that there may be strep or staph infection down inside the facial acne bumps. For this reason, your doctor may choose to change your antibiotic to one which will knock out these bacteria.

Cosmetics and Acne

Q: I am a 38-year-old with two children, and my acne is worse now than when I was a teenager or when I was pregnant. I was always under the impression that skin problems of this sort would disappear as a woman got older. Not true?

A: Unfortunately, that's not true. As I've said before, acne is a disease of an ever older age group, a fact which has distressed many of us in dermatology.

We believe there are two general reasons for this. First, we have tried over the years to increase patient awareness of what can be done for acne so that many men and women now consult dermatologists earlier for a few bumps rather than put up with them until they scar and go away on their own. It's this patient concern which has brought about the demand for ever more effective acne medications.

Second, cosmetic industry leaders, while doing what they can to protect against cosmetic-induced acne, have not completely succeeded. That is, most cosmetics are still inducing acne. This situation is compounded for older women since our looks-conscious society demands a continued youthful appearance. The result often is an increasing use of cosmetics to mask minor flaws. Then the cosmetics themselves can cause a plugging of oil glands, or some change in the secretion of oil, which we see later as "acne cosmetica" (acne induced and sustained by cosmetics). The following letter will demonstrate how very common it is for women to want to cover their acne blemishes.

Q: I am disgusted! I have had acne cosmetica since I was 28 and my medical doctor has always told me that he could not cure acne, and that there was nothing I could do but live with it. I've heard you mention a makeup that is used in covering birthmarks, and I wondered if I could use this to cover my bumps.

A: Your true problem is twofold. First, you're not doing much in terms of a treatment regimen to help clear your skin; second, acne cosmetica must be treated by cessation of the offending cosmetic and substitution of one or more which do not usually cause acne.

The birthmark makeup you're talking about is called Covermark (discussed in Chapter 3). While Covermark will successfully and safely cover almost any flat spot on the skin, the one thing with which it has difficulty is a bump on the skin. As Dr. Marsh always told me, "Smooth, unmade-up skin looks better than made-up bumpy skin!"

However, the Covermark cosmetic system is reportedly not acnegenic. The problem is one of difficulty in application, because the Covermark system requires extra steps which preclude one from using any topical medications prescribed by a dermatologist.

Acne cosmetica is a very severe and widespread problem. It was discovered when researchers were testing the inner ears of rabbits for the irritant potential of cosmetics. Some of their results were not irritation, but whiteheads and blackheads on the rabbit ear skin. So substances such as cold creams and makeup are now used as the *test* substances to *produce* experimental acne in which new therapeutic medications may be tried!

DERMALERT

Cosmetics are one of the leading causes of acne in this country.

Now I'm not trying to kill off the cosmetic industry. I think cosmetics are a prime requisite in our society today, and I would not ask women to go without them, since there are now systems which can be used which do not induce new acne. The best is the one made by Cosmedics Research Laboratory: the Dermage system.

This system originated from a dermatologist named Dr. Gloria Graham, one of the world's leading acne therapists and cryosurgeons, in practice in Wilson, North Carolina, jointly with Rachel Lubritz, wife of a dermatologist and prominent businesswoman, who later became president of Dermage. The initial testing was done by Dr. Albert M. Kligman at the Ivy Research Labs, and the original product formulation was compiled by George Fiedler, DSC. This relatively new cosmetic system has been investigated thoroughly to make sure that it does not cause acne. Each and every ingredient, as well as the final products in the Dermage line, has been tested on humans and on rabbit ears to make sure that it does not cause acne.

The Dermage system has the further advantage of two different lines of makeup, both of which are hypoallergenic (of course, acne is not an allergy, but the hypoallergenicity of the Dermage system helps with other conditions, such as contact dermatitis or topical skin allergy). The first is called the Mauve line and is designed for women with acne problems and/or excess oil. It can be used very effectively in teenagers with acne difficulties, because acne medicines can be applied to the face beneath the Dermage cosmetics, which are applied by a "patting on" motion. And that's the real point. Dermage is a surface cosmetic system, pure and simple. It was never designed to be rubbed into the skin.

The other line, called the Pearl line, has built-in moisturizers. This is for older women who are starting to lose oil gland output and who require slight moisturization. Occasionally, we'll have an acne patient who is getting too dry on her topical medications and we can switch her back and forth from Mauve to Pearl in order to recover some needed skin moisture.

DERMALERT

Acne is not an allergy. Hypoallergenic makeups do not help acne just because they say they're hypoallergenic. It's far more important for cosmetics which are expected to be used in acne and complexion problems to state that they are *noncomedogenic*.

Until the Dermage cosmetic system came along, my standard axiom was "A little makeup, a little paint, sure makes acne where it ain't!" So if you have any tendency toward acne, and if you want to give yourself a fighting chance, you should use the Dermage system. Research shows that to do otherwise may be gambling with the only face you've got. Ask your dermatologist about Dermage. Currently, it's only available through a physician's office. If your dermatologist can't tell you about it, call or write the company at:

Dermage Cosmedics Research Laboratories, Inc.
601 Harper Street
Wilson, North Carolina 27893
(919) 243-3212

Other companies which have excellent nonacnegenic lines are Clinique, Allercreme, Almay, and Elizabeth Arden.

Hormones—The Match That Lights the Acne Fire

Q: I recently had a hysterectomy and I feel embarrassed to ask my doctor about my skin. I am breaking out on my neck, face, and ears quite severely, and it's driving me crazy, since I'm already 39 years old. I feel like a teenager. What can I do?

A: You don't tell me whether or not your doctor removed your ovaries when he performed your hysterectomy. Often, however, that is the case, and that would result in a drastic drop in the amount of estrogen in your system (your ovaries make estrogen). Estrogen, as you know, is a female hormone which can combat acne. Therefore, when your ovaries were removed, if indeed they were, you had a sudden decrease in the amount of estrogen in your system. This allowed your small amount of male hormones (androgens) to stimulate your oil glands and cause new acne. We often see this happen, albeit somewhat more slowly, around the time of natural menopause, when a few bumps come on very gradually.

DERMALERT

Surgical menopause (the removal of ovaries) can cause a rapid onset of acne.

You should know, however, that there are some diseases which manifest themselves first by a low-grade case of acne. Some of these diseases are endocrine in nature and involve such problems as ovarian cysts or pituitary or even adrenal difficulties. If your doctor did not remove your ovaries when your uterus was removed and your acne persists, have your doctor check you for endocrine gland problems.

The treatment of acne in your age group is basically the same as the treatment in teenagers except that you will not need as much drying in order to clear. Often antibiotics are necessary to suppress the outbreak of new lesions. That's where the drug tetracycline comes in very handy. It can slow down or stop the appearance of new bumps by preventing the rotting of oil in the sebaceous glands within the skin.

DERMALERT

If acne appears suddenly at any time in your life, it can indicate the presence of an endocrine (hormone-secreting) gland problem.

Antibiotics

Antibiotics have assumed a major role in the treatment of acne, and many of my questions from new acne patients involve the use of antibiotics.

Q: I'm on tetracycline for my complexion. But I have trouble remembering to take it, since my doctor says it must be taken on an empty stomach. Got any suggestions?

A: Try to tie the taking of your medicine with some other action repeated in your daily routine. For one of my patients, I recommended he store the tablet bottle in his slipper near his bed at night, and keep a glass of water on his nightstand. When he awakened each morning, his foot struck the bottle as he put his slippers on, causing him to remember to take his pill. It worked like a charm! Of course, you could *not* use this trick if you have small children at home. Naturally, all medicines must be kept out of their reach.

If you're on a medicine which may be taken close to meals, I often advise attaching one's toothbrush to the medicine bottle with a rubber band. Then, each time you brush, you'll be reminded about your medicine. This is, of course, contingent upon brushing your teeth after eating!

Q: Why is it important to take this antibiotic on an empty stomach?

A: As your doctor has already told you, tetracycline should be taken on an empty stomach as much as possible. Most forms of tetracycline are greatly affected by meals, especially by the calcium in food. That's generally why milk is to be avoided during acne therapy. But it's even more important that the directions for taking one's medicine be clearly written and clearly understood. A patient of mine named Teresa very adequately illustrates this point. Teresa came in with small papular acne, i.e., mostly small red bumps. This is usually the easiest type of acne to clear, and it usually clears beautifully on tetracycline capsules. Teresa was instructed to take one capsule three times a day, and on her prescription I wrote "one hour a.c. or two hours p.c." This means "one hour before meals or two hours after meals." Teresa was using her topical medicines faithfully and was taking her capsules, three a day, but was not clearing. Her bumps kept getting worse instead of better even when I increased the dose of tetracycline to four a day.

On her third visit, we were both fairly disturbed with the continual outbreak of new spots, and Teresa asked me if there was any special way to take the medicine. I asked, "Aren't you taking it one hour before meals or two hours after, as I suggested?"

"Did you say, 'before or after meals'?" she asked.

"Yes, as I had written on the prescription," I said, rather impatiently.

"But my bottle says nothing about the time I'm supposed to take it!"

"Do you have it with you?" I asked.

Her hand dipped into her purse and emerged with the bottle. The label read, "Take one capsule three times a day."

"Is that all they had to say about when you should take it?" I asked.

"Yes," she said, "so I've been taking it *with* meals!"

Now we had the answer to Teresa's antibiotic dilemma. When I instructed her to take it on an empty stomach, she started to clear rapidly.

DERMALERT

Tetracycline should always be taken on an empty stomach. This permits much better absorption, and you actually get an effect from the medicine you purchased.

The exception to this empty stomach rule is a drug called *minocycline*, a very effective tetracycline derivative which you need not take on an empty stomach. One problem with minocycline, however, is that it's much more expensive than regular tetracycline. In fact, we usually reserve it for difficult cases of acne because of its cost. However, in cases where patients cannot get themselves to take tetracycline on an empty stomach, it is very easy to take minocycline because they can pop a capsule at mealtime.

The prohibition against food with regular tetracycline has caused some occasional problems. Jennifer, a 13-year-old with acne, called me in a panic in the middle of the night stating that she just knew that she was going to die because of the tetracycline she took! "Had she overdosed?" I wondered. Tearful, she said that she had accidentally taken her tetracycline with food and the label specifically said never to do this. She was afraid she would have some terrible reaction. I reassured her that taking the medicine with food just slowed down its absorption and did not cause any toxic effects. Jennifer returned to bed much calmer than when she had called.

If you're on regular tetracycline, you might remember the bottle-in-the-slipper trick mentioned before (provided you don't have any little kids around the house). Also, taking it at nighttime before bed usually provides you with a fairly empty stomach (unless you're a midnight snacker).

Q: I've been on tetracyline for two years trying to get my acne cleared. I am an 18-year-old girl, and I'm concerned about how long I can take this medicine safely.

A: This question is very important because of the scare implanted in laypersons during the early days of antibiotic therapy. At that time, lay audiences were told that use of antibiotics for a long term would cause a "resistance" to them which would preclude their use in infections at a later date. Actually the group of antibiotics used most often in acne, that is, the tetracyclines, are found to be some of the safest drugs ever invented. While there are side effects, these are uncommon in actual practice.

The chief side effect, usually occurring in women on doses of 500 to 1000 milligrams and more per day, is vaginitis. Regular vaginal bacteria are suppressed by the antibiotic and yeasts overgrow. Then an itchy discharge can develop which is quite annoying, but this does not always mean that the patient has to stop the medication. In many cases, since the face is the "window with which one greets the world," it is absolutely necessary to keep up the antibiotic, and in these cases, we usually prescribe vaginal clotrimazole tablets once or twice a week to prevent yeast infection. There are many other drugs which can perform this function, and your doctor may have another preference. But don't give up hope just because you get an episode of vaginitis. It's a problem which can be very adequately controlled.

Various other side effects of taking tetracycline include nausea and, with minocycline, occasional dizzy spells. Your own dermatologist can brief you on other problems associated with tetracycline in the treatment of acne.

Antibiotics and "The Pill"

Recent reports from Australia indicate that tetracycline occasionally diminishes the contraceptive effect of the low-dose birth control pill. Therefore, if you are on the pill, ask your physician whether you should be on tetracycline simultaneously. If your physician doesn't want you on the two together, he or she may want to ask your dermatologist to switch you to erythromycin, which has much the same type of activity that tetracycline has in acne, but which is only about one-half to two-thirds as effective when given internally. One advantage is that erythromycin usually does not cause vaginitis.

DERMALERT

If you're on a low-dose birth control pill (the "mini-pill") and if you're under treatment for acne, ask your gynecologist or dermatologist whether or not there is a risk of pregnancy with the antibiotic you're taking.

Q: Speaking of the birth control pill (BCP), I'm on one and my acne is getting worse. Any connection?

A: Yes. As you may know, oral contraceptives are combinations of estrogens and progestins. While the estrogen component is not acne-causing, the progestin in most pills is broken down by the body into a substance which has androgenic (male hormone) effects. This makes acne worse.

There are, however, several types of BCPs which are not usually thought to make acne worse. In these BCPs, the progestin is

metabolized to an estrogenic substance which may actually help
clear acne.

Ask your physician which of these so-called estrogen-domi-
nant types is preferred for you. Your doctor will usually be glad
to change types if you haven't had any pill-related problems. For
most BCPs, the pill + skin = acne. Ask your doctor for one which
will not satisfy this equation.

Antibiotics and Teeth

Q: My 13-year-old son has been on tetracycline for some time
and I am concerned about the possible staining of his teeth on
this antibiotic. Is it likely to happen to him and how long does it
take?

A: This is another one of the really misplaced bits of information which gets planted in the lay literature without adequate
explanation. Mothers, fathers, and adolescent patients ask this
question repeatedly. Tetracycline can cause tooth staining, and
even malformation of the teeth, if it's taken before the age of 8.
This can also happen to the fetus of a woman who is pregnant,
if she takes tetracycline. Therefore, physicians who prescribe tetracycline are *very* cautious not to give it to young children or
pregnant mothers. If neither of these conditions applies, that is,
if you're not under the age of 8, and if you're not pregnant, there
can be no dental problems with tetracycline.

DERMALERT

Tetracycline can cause fetal tooth staining and faulty
enamel development if a mother takes it while she is
pregnant or if a child takes it before the age of 8.

An exception to the rule about tetracycline tooth staining (concerning the drug minocycline) is discussed in the November 22,
1985, *Journal of the American Medical Association*. Dr. Gary L. Peck,
the chief researcher in the development of Accutane, and his
fellow researchers discovered that four patients out of seventy-

two surveyed showed some degree of tooth staining, even though the medicine had been given during adolescence. These researchers postulate that the binding of minocycline with iron may be responsible for the staining. Sadly, the stains do not seem to fade after time.

The general recommendation in regard to minocycline would change somewhat in light of this newest information. I'll still treat severe acne patients with the drug, but I'll warn them about the tooth staining properties of the medicine, and stop it at the first sign of darkening of the enamel of the teeth.

A recent study concerning tetracycline was reviewed at the American Academy of Dermatology meeting in December 1981. A large group of patients on tetracycline for acne were followed carefully over several years, and no problems arose in the adolescents' health, either by physical examination or by lab studies. Of course, as with any prescription medicine, your dermatologist will want to see adolescent patients from time to time, to make sure they are on the right dose of the medication and that all their topical medications are being used correctly.

Miscellaneous Questions About Acne

Q: I'm 27 years old, and every month I get two or three red bumps on either my chin or neck. I don't have much of an acne problem because I keep my face well cleansed. My problem is very difficult, though, since I get it monthly. Can you tell me something I can do to get rid of this period-related problem?

A: Often, period-related acne is well controlled by increasing the amount of internal medicine your physician has prescribed about five to seven days before periods. This should be done *only* on your dermatologist's advice, however, because some medicines cannot be adjusted this way.

More important, you should know that acne is only helped minimally by facial cleansing. It is not dirt which is responsible for acne; it's a problem deep down in the oil glands. So washing frequently helps only insofar as it removes dead skin cells and surface oil. Washing too vigorously or too frequently can even *cause* new acne, a problem now dubbed "acne mechanica."

Q: Is acne contagious? Both my parents had it.

A: Absolutely not. There is no contagious form of acne with a possible exception of the rare case of antibiotic-resistant acne. In this type, a real bacterial infection develops deep in the oil glands. This is treatable by changing to an antibiotic which kills whatever bacteria are currently infecting the lesions.

The fact that both your parents had severe acne and you do, too, bears out the generally accepted theory that if each of your parents had bad acne you have about an 80 percent chance of having it also.

Q: My little girl is only 9 years old and is getting some early bumps on her face. But she is not even having periods yet! Is this possible?

A: Yes, and it's very, very common. Acne often heralds the onset of menstrual periods by as much as two years in children.

Q: My 15-year-old daughter has acne bumps on her face and shoulders and was told to change pillow slips nightly and use clean towels and washcloths every time she washes, but it has not helped. What can we use that is not too expensive and still can help her acne?

A: Changing pillowcases and towels will not aid in the resolution of her acne. Again, this old saw that acne is due to dirt is completely untrue. However, the sulfur medications sometimes used at night tend to flake off on the pillow and it may be necessary for that reason to change her pillowcase, but in general she can use her own judgment with regard to this.

Unfortunately, acne care tends to be moderately expensive. And the age-old adage that you get what you pay for may certainly apply in acne therapy, since some of the medicines used are quite expensive. But they are also quite effective. You might ask your dermatologist for samples of medications he or she intends to use with your daughter to cut down on costs. Many dermatologists supply their patients with samples, and it certainly never hurts to ask.

Attacking the Oil Factories with Retinoids— The New Vitamin A

Q: I have really oily skin and I have tried everything to help, including antiseptic cleansers and so forth. Is there anything I can use to get rid of the oiliness? I have very few pimples.

A: The oiliness of facial skin has always been a problem. Some people actually secrete so much oil that even after wiping it off they are able to see it visibly reappear within five minutes on the nose.

Until recently there was nothing which would really decrease oil secretion. Most dermatologists felt that it was important to remove it, but there was no way to shut it down from the inside.

However, there has recently been developed a class of drugs known as the *retinoids* which holds tremendous promise for acne patients with excess oil secretion problems. While retinoids have been in use in Europe for several years, they have only recently been released by the Food and Drug Administration (FDA) for use in acne here in this country.

Retinoids are chemically bent forms of vitamin A and appear to work in several ways. First, they shut down the production of oil in the oil gland and shrink its size. They also decrease inflammation and have some antibacterial effect. But their prime function in acne is to correct the basic defect which causes plugs down inside the oil glands. No one yet knows exactly how this works, but these drugs, when used by trained dermatologists, are extremely effective. For the first time in acne therapy we may be able to use the word "cure" for up to 94 percent of those people with the most severe type of acne, nodulocystic acne. It's this kind which causes most of the scars on youngsters.

Dr. Gary Peck's study at the National Institutes of Health showed dramatic improvement in acne bumps after treatment with a retinoid called 13-cis-retinoid, or brand name Accutane. The medicine is taken by mouth once or twice a day; over about five months, the acne process gradually comes to a halt.

Should your physician choose not to use the drug in your case (see why below), there are other things you may do to help your oiliness problem. Among these are the topically applied form of vitamin A called Retin-A. Retin-A appears to have some of the same effects topically of retinoids given internally in the treatment of acne. However, as I've previously mentioned, it can be irritating, and I use it less frequently on my patients because of the redness it produces.

Benzoyl peroxides also can dry the skin sufficiently so that it looks as though very little oil is being secreted. Sometimes it's necessary to use a 10% or even a 20% specially made benzoyl peroxide for this purpose. Benzoyl peroxide can irritate the skin too, so be sure to ask your doctor which strength is right for your skin type.

DERMALERT

The tide may be turning in our favor in acne therapy. With Accutane, it's possible to shut down even cystic acne and avoid the nuisance of topically applied medications.

Q: Accutane sounds terrific! Who can take it? Are there any complications?

A: Whoa! Not everyone can take Accutane. It's only for the 5 percent of acne patients who have the chronic cystic, recalcitrant, scarring kind of acne. And there are complications, such as extreme dryness, chapping, headaches, fatigue, lip irritation, eye dryness, joint and muscle aches, and elevation of fats (cholesterol and triglycerides) in the blood. This necessitates frequent lab tests at the start of therapy.

The medicine is also very expensive.

Q: You stated that retinoids were a type of vitamin A. If I take vitamin A by mouth, will my acne improve?

A: For years, dermatologists have prescribed vitamin A with very little success. Dr. Al Kligman, noted acne specialist from Pennsylvania, states that vitamin A will have some of the effects of Accutane if given in near toxic doses. The problem is that one risks side effects of vitamin A even when treating acne with moderate doses. Vitamin A is one of the fat-soluble vitamins, stored in the liver. Caucasians who first went to Alaska and the Arctic region got very sick when they ate polar bear meat if they included in their diet the *liver* of the bear. It has such incredible concentrations of vitamin A that it is poisonous.

Q: Well, then, why isn't Accutane toxic?

A: Accutane is not stored in the liver, and it is rapidly excreted. But it's extremely important *not* to take regular vitamin A if your dermatologist is giving you Accutane. They'll occasionally interact, making each one stronger.

Q: How about the effect of Accutane on pregnancy?

A: Retinoids can cause defective fetuses in rats and humans. It's absolutely mandatory that pregnant women *not* take it, and that women taking Accutane not *get* pregnant while taking it.

Q: Can Accutane be used for anything else?

A: The amazing thing about the retinoids is that their salutary effects are not limited to the treatment of acne. There are many diseases of excess scaliness of the skin which they appear to help marvelously, and, amazingly enough, there are retinoid effects which may hold great promise for everyone's future. Among these is their anticancer effect. Retinoids, when given to experimental animals, appear to reverse precancerous changes in epithelial or skinlike body tissues of bladder and breast. In fact, there has been a remarkable inhibition of breast cancer in certain types of rats who get this disease with incredible facility. If this turns out to be the case, many may get retinoids in the future to reverse precancerous changes. Note that FDA approval for Accutane is only for its use in severe nodulocystic acne.

DERMALERT

Vitamin A therapy is not completely harmless. It's possible to get very ill on regular vitamin A if large doses are taken for acne.

Q: My son is on Accutane for cystic acne. How long will he have to take it?

A: Taking the medicine for four or five months often acts as a functional *cure* in recalcitrant cystic acne, and this effect persists even after the medicine is stopped. Some kids have to be treated a second time, but most clear progressively and have no further problems.

Nose "Blackheads"

Q: My 8-year-old daughter has a bad case of blackheads on her nose. I know it's not dirt because I wash her face every night. She also washes it in the morning. Her skin cannot be that oily, can it?

A: As a matter of fact, it can! The nose is a characteristic place for blackheads to occur, but most children of your daughter's age do not have true blackheads. Most of them have simple dots at the top of columns of oil which lead down into the oil glands on the nose. These are usually quite deep but are not the massively obstructed oil glands represented in blackheads. It's often possible to squeeze the nasal skin gently and coax these tiny dots to the surface where they can be wiped off. Certainly she should not be doing her own acne surgery, but this can show you the type of lesion or spot that these are.

Treatment is very difficult. The black dot is *not* dirt, but a pigment called melanin picked up from the surrounding skin cells. All the washing in the world will help this only slightly. Agents like the potent forms of benzoyl peroxide, which I've already mentioned, can help lighten these lesions chronically. However, the tiny dots (even in the middle-aged patient) are usually not visible at a conversational distance, so the sufferer need not feel self-conscious about them.

The Sun and Acne

Q: I used a sunlamp several years ago and caused a rash of zits. Is this possible?

A: Sunlight usually helps acne, but reports over the last several years indicate that *intense* sunlight or sunlamp exposure can actually induce new bumps. This is becoming more and more a problem because of the desire of adolescents for a dark suntan.

Some of these kids come in with a tremendous crop of acne lesions just *because* of excess sun exposure.

Keep in mind that the sun actually damages the skin. This damage consists not only of wrinkles but of the induction of pre-malignant spots and actual malignant skin cancers. Most dermatologists do not prescribe sunlight for the treatment of acne. The major exception is in widespread acne of the back and trunk in which phototherapy is a very useful adjunct.

My mentor in dermatology, Dr. Glenn Marsh, is very fond of telling a story about one patient, a young woman named Stacy, who showed up in his office with the most incredible case of acne that he had ever seen. Stacy had terrible nodulocystic and bleeding lesions on the nape of her neck, all over her face, the front of her neck, and the chest all the way to the beltline, front and back. In short, she was a total mess!

"What in the world happened to you?" the dermatologist said.

"Not much, just a little sun bathing," she replied.

"Did you put anything on your skin?"

"Well, I found this new preparation my friend had recommended which gave me a fantastic rapid tan," she replied.

"Well, what was it?" he asked, "Essence of Acne?"

"Nope. Sheer, fresh, 10-W-30 motor oil!" she exclaimed.

He had no problem figuring out that it wasn't entirely the sun that had caused her acne. Motor oil on the skin of a human being can cause acne almost anywhere!

DERMALERT

Not only sun but suntan lotions which are not approved by your dermatologist can cause new acne bumps. Ask your dermatologist about the correct lotion to use to avoid sun damage and also avoid acne.

Sulfa versus Sulfur

Q: I've always been allergic to sulfa and my doctor gave me an acne medication which has sulfur as its base. I have had some drying with the medication, and occasionally some stinging, and wondered if this medication is doing this because of a possible similar reaction to it.

A: You may very well be confusing the words "sulf*a*" and "sulf*ur*." Sulfa is an antibiotic given internally for various infections, though allergic reactions can develop to it.

While allergic reactions can also (on rare occasions) develop to sulfur used topically, the two drugs are not related and should not cross-react in any way. The sulfur that you may be using on your skin is a drying agent which can indeed cause stinging and itching. But this is usually not an allergic reaction, and decreasing the strength of the medicine, or the frequency of its application, can alleviate this problem altogether.

DERMALERT

Sulfa and sulfur are two different compounds. *Sulfur* is a topically applied drying agent used in acne, and *sulfa* is an internal antibiotic.

X-ray Therapy

Q: As a 30-year-old, I had quite severe acne which was treated several times with x-ray therapy. Later I had a benign brain tumor removed after a long battle with seizures. Do you think my x-ray therapy caused my brain tumor?

A: The neurosurgeons to whom I've spoken have very much doubted that the two are at all related. However, your neurosurgeon should be consulted with any questions you have about the tumor problem.

Your question brings up a very important note about past acne therapy. It has been known ever since the turn of the century that x-ray therapy can decrease the size of oil glands and help acne. However, researchers found some twenty to thirty years later that x-ray therapy given for acne can cause problems with growths in the thyroid gland in the neck, especially when the neck was not shielded during the x-ray procedure. So most dermatologists are recommending that any patients who have ever been treated with x-ray for acne have a yearly check of their thyroid with a physical examination and certain laboratory tests so that their internist or endocrinologist can follow their thyroid status carefully.

DERMALERT

X-ray therapy for acne has been related to thyroid cancer. If anyone you know has ever had x-ray therapy for acne, they should be checked regularly by an internist so that any potential thyroid problems can be detected early.

These days x-ray therapy for acne has been largely abandoned. My own opinion is that, even though it works, the hazards of x-rays are too great to allow its use in acne therapy.

Zinc

Q: I've heard a lot of talk about zinc in acne therapy. Is this a hoax?

A: Several years ago reports indicated that zinc therapy in acne resulted in early clearing of acne bumps. So most of us jumped on the early bandwagon and gave our patients moderate to high doses of zinc, and then stood back to observe the quick improvement which had been described. However, we succeeded only in nauseating some of our adolescents. Zinc didn't help acne a bit.

I've noticed that the health food stores are two to three years behind in their recommendations on what *they* think will cure acne. They are currently recommending zinc, and since they can't follow their "patients" as we do in dermatology, they probably will take a lot longer to notice its nausea-producing side effects.

Acne is *not* a disease related to vitamin deficiency. (In this country, it's very hard to even find someone who's vitamin-deficient. Even most junk food these days is crammed full of vitamins so that it's nearly impossible to get short-changed in this regard.) Don't bother pursuing acne therapy with vitamins and trace elements.

Shots for Acne

Q: I get huge hollow knots on my facial skin that my dermatologist wants to inject with a substance. What is he going to inject, and should I let him do it?

A: The huge knots on your face are acne cysts. They are spots of tremendous inflammation which your doctor is attempting to decrease by injecting medicine right into them.

The medicine he wants to use is a type of cortisone, usually one called *triamcinolone*. Triamcinolone in small quantities inside the cyst can make it shrink until the body's natural defenses reabsorb the cystic sac. While you should certainly discuss these injections with your doctor, they are usually very desirable in order to decrease the healing time of these scarring lesions.

You should know, however, that there is a risk of atrophy in the area below the cyst injected with this material. This means that the fat layer beneath the cyst is caused to thin out at least temporarily in some cases. This can leave a small sunken spot for a few weeks. This is why most of us choose to use a very low strength medicine that may have to be repeatedly injected every three to four weeks. Usually this low-strength dilution of triamcinolone will not cause the fat atrophy. However, the medicine Accutane sounds very appropriate for you (see above) and you might discuss it with your doctor.

Q: If the dermatologist can inject medicine into cysts and get them to heal faster, why can't he do the same for ordinary zits?

A: Ordinary acne bumps have no cavity within them to speak of so that there is no room to put the steroid material. Any attempt to inject a small papule or bump usually results in leakage of the medicine out into the surrounding skin, causing more problems with sunken spots.

DERMALERT

Large cystic lesions in acne can usually be healed very quickly by the injection of cortisone right into the cysts.

In this chapter, I've discussed active acne and the many treatments for it. In the next chapter I'll tell you the secrets of fixing acne scars if they have already occurred.

8

—

Restoring Acne-Scarred Skin

You now know a lot about what causes acne and about what can be done when it develops. But what if you found this book too late? What if *your* cystic acne occurred before we *had* Accutane and powerful antibiotics? Take a look around and you'll see dozens of ex-acne sufferers for whom our dermatological miracles came too late. Does that mean it's too late to help your scarring? Absolutely not!

There are several methods developed in the last six years that you and your doctor can choose from to resurface your scars. Usually a combination of dermatological and plastic surgical techniques are used. Many dermatologists and dermatologic surgeons can perform the whole restoration process, so ask your doctor—talking it over long and hard is the *only* way. Not all techniques will work for everybody, and it's important that you know what you're in for.

Take dermabrasion, for example. It's a major procedure fraught with complications, and sometimes a single dermabrasion won't do the whole job. Let's take a closer look.

The Dermabrasion Dilemma

Q: I had a dermabrasion in 1977 at the age of 27. The doctor said it would help surface marks but that another dermabrasion might be necessary to remove deeper marks. Is it a normal procedure to have two operations?

A: Dermabrasion, or facial planing, is used to recontour and smoothen the surface of the skin. It is a procedure which is not to be taken lightly, since it causes a tremendous amount of temporary disability (weeping, pain, crusting, and possible secondary infection) and some long-term disabilities (several months or longer of altered skin color, sun sensitivity, and possible further scarring). In this procedure, the dermatologist or plastic surgeon briefly freezes the skin, and then sands off the upper layers with a small diamond-coated wheel or brush. This is done under general or local anesthesia.

The sanding is continued until tiny bleeding points are reached in the skin. This indicates that the proper depth for scar removal has been reached. Depending on the type of scarring you have, one such operation may suffice; if the scars are deep, two operations may be needed. While there are hazards associated with dermabrasion, such as infection, variation in skin color, and even scarring induced by the operation, it is, in general, a safe procedure when done by skilled hands. It is not always possible, of course, to sand out every scar with the first procedure or even with the second one. You should be sure to discuss all the pros and cons of this treatment with your dermatologist or plastic surgeon.

DERMALERT

Dermabrasion, or skin planing, can produce scarring of its own in some instances, as well as variations in skin pigment. As with any procedure, discussion of it with your surgeon will clarify any possible complications.

Q: Could the second dermabrasion be performed in the surgeon's office on an outpatient basis to avoid the high hospital cost?

A: Very frequently dermabrasions are done in the offices of dermatologists and plastic surgeons. This can avoid the high cost of hospitalization, but the procedure itself is fairly expensive, ranging from $1,000 to $2,500, depending on the surgeon and on the size of the area that must be abraded. Most dermabrasions are full face, because if there is any pigment or texture change in the skin, it's more desirable to have the entire face look the same.

Q: Will hospitalization insurance cover my dermabrasion costs?

A: If the dermabrasion is done to treat active acne (as is sometimes the case) most insurance policies will reimburse you. However, even if the policy does not reimburse you, dermabrasion, like other cosmetic procedures, can function as a tax deduction. Talk to your physician and your tax adviser and health insurance company concerning this *before* you make plans.

Q: Can dermabrasion remove all scars and leave some degree of smooth skin?

A: Nothing can restore the skin to its "preacne" quality. But dermabrasion, combined sometimes with chemical peels and other rehabilitative efforts, which we will discuss, can result in a better appearance.

Q: Could a face-lift provide more desirable results than a dermabrasion?

A: If you have significant wrinkling due to age and sun changes, a combined procedure of a face-lift and dermabrasion may help you to a greater degree.

Dermabrasion should not be regarded as a cure-all for scarring or any other problem. There are complications with the procedure, and everyone who undergoes it should be fully aware of these complications. The following stories amply demonstrate some of the problems that can be incurred. Be sure you fully inquire about complications before you undergo *any* surgical procedure.

Q: Some years ago I had a dermabrasion on my face for acne scars and I had such a violent reaction that they could only do one planing. Originally they said I would need three. Apparently as a result of the planing, I have indented white scars on both cheeks. I am in the public eye, so you can imagine the trauma that this has caused. We felt the results of the dermabrasion would be worth the pain and expense, but now things are actually worse. I am 64 years old, but even at this age it would be great to find something that would help to cover the scars.

Q: In March 1980 I underwent a dermabrasion for my entire facial area. Prior to the operation I was informed that there would be little, if any, pain involved. Since I was fair-complexioned, the possibility of discoloration was not a concern; I was supposed to notice a marked overall improvement of my facial areas since the doctor who was to perform the operation did not consider my particular facial scarring that serious.

Armed with this information, I subjected myself to the most painful experience of my life. My face is now discolored and the pigment is lost forever. Not only did the dermabrasion fail to improve any part of my face, but it left scarring and one very deep and discolored area that I did not have previously on my upper lip. Most of my face now looks worse. My reason for writing you is that since your television appearance and subsequent commentary on the newer methods of treatment for acne and scarring, I have regained some degree of hope. Please let others know about my experience.

A: I think these tragic stories speak for themselves. In this regard dermabrasion, as I have said before, should be approached with your eyes open as both a patient and a consumer.

Collagen Implants

Q: Can you furnish me with more information about the product designed to raise the center of a scar and even out the top layer of skin?

A: The remarkable stuff you are asking about is called Zyderm injectable collagen implant. This material is a thick gel produced by chemically breaking up leather into its component parts. The process makes it very similar to human collagen, the support network for the skin. That's the part of the skin which actually holds it together, just like the leather in a leather coat.

Zyderm was tested with thousands of patients for several years prior to its approval by the FDA and its release in the spring of 1981.

The substance of collagen can be equated to a group of small molecular bricks which cement themselves together under the skin when the correct body temperature and environment are reached.

Zyderm should be used only by dermatologists specially trained by the Collagen Corporation. Some—not all—acne scars respond beautifully to it. The material is injected below saucerlike, gently rolling acne scars, and elevates the center of the scar, thus making shadowing in the scar a lot less noticeable. The scars do not actually go away but their visibility is in most instances greatly reduced.

Treatment with Zyderm for acne scars or any other scars consists of two steps. The first is a test injection: a small amount is injected under the skin of the forearm and allowed to sit in place for a month to detect any possible allergies. If, after a month, the dermatologist finds no sign of redness or firmness which might indicate allergy, then the injections of the scars can begin.

DERMALERT

There are occasional very rare reactions to Zyderm when it is injected on the face, even though the skin test was negative. Be sure you ask your physician about this complication prior to injection therapy with Zyderm injectable collagen implant.

There are, however, several groups of patients who cannot be injected with Zyderm. These are patients who have autoimmune diseases, a type of allergic reaction to one or more of the body's own organs. Chief among these is rheumatoid arthritis. Others include Crohn's disease, Graves' disease, discoid lupus, systemic lupus, Sjögren's syndrome, ulcerative colitis, Reiter's syndrome, psoriatic arthritis, progressive systemic sclerosis, polymyositis, and polyarteritis.

DERMALERT

Patients with rheumatoid arthritis or any related autoimmune diseases should not get Zyderm collagen
implants. Also there are other diseases which preclude injection of this new substance.

Collagen Injection

Q: On the average, how many injections of collagen are needed
to smoothen scars, and over what length of time?

A: While the specific number of treatments is determined by
the results after the first injection, it is possible to say in general
that most acne patients need at least three and sometimes four
or five injections to maximally correct scars. After the one-month
waiting period to determine if the skin test is negative, injections
can be performed every two weeks until the therapy is completed.

Q: Can many scars be treated in one session? How long does
it take?

A: Yes, multiple scars are usually treated in a single session.
Often, I do an entire side of the face in an acne-scarred patient
and sometimes the entire facial surface. There is really no limit
to the number of lesions which can be treated in each session,
but, practically speaking, one or two milliliters of material is the
usual dose injected at one sitting.

Q: Would the benefits of collagen treatment be altered in any
way if one were to have subsequent skin peelings?

A: Since Zyderm is injected into the skin, there is no reason
at all to suspect that subsequent skin peelings or dermabrasions
would affect the treatments in any way. Many dermatologists and
plastic surgeons combine procedures.

Q: How much does Zyderm cost?

A: This depends on the number of scars you have to rehabilitate, but the material is quite expensive. It ranges in cost from
about $150 to $200 per milliliter, and one milliliter can often treat
between ten and fifteen scars depending upon their size. You

should realize, however, that possible subsequent injections may be needed, and the cost for the Zyderm is usually exclusive of the dermatologist's office visit fee or the fee you pay to utilize the dermatologist's skills in making these very exacting injections.

Therefore, you can see that a person who has fifteen slightly depressed acne scars in the face and who needs one milliliter of treatment for three or four visits could pay $450 to $800 for the therapy. Costs vary, of course, and you should consult your dermatologist for an estimate.

Q: How long-lasting is the Zyderm material?

A: As yet we do not know, since the material has not been in use long enough. But based on collagen replacement studies, there is no reason at all to suspect that it may not be present for six months to two years after the initial injection.

Since collagen is continually replaced and not just eliminated from the skin, it may be possible for the newly injected collagen to be renewed with one's *own* skin collagen rather than just to be eliminated. If this turns out to be the case, collagen may be a semipermanent treatment. But the company does say that periodic touch-ups or reinjections will be necessary. In my experience, most patients need these yearly.

Q: Can collagen implants be used to treat areas of multiple scars or only single isolated scars?

A: Zyderm is effective in single and multiple scars. The medicine is supplied in various quantities and in three different consistencies, so that your dermatologist can select the one right for you in terms of the amount needed. The medicine works best for the types of multiple rolling scars we see after cystic acne, but not as well in the tiny punctate, sharply demarcated, ice-pick type scars we see in some kids who have had scarring acne.

The newer Zyplast implant is much denser, and can correct deep defects in the skin of acne patients and patients left with sunken spots due to disease or surgery. This type of collagen is injected *below* the skin.

Punch Excision of Scars

Q: Are Zyderm collagen implant treatments the best treatment for chicken pox scars?

A: Chicken pox scars have a fairly sharp edge which makes the elevation of them quite difficult. Often these are best treated by plastic surgical intervention with dermabrasion ("skin sanding") or actual excision, or cutting out of the scar.

Some skin surgeons prefer to cut out the scar with a small punch biopsy, or cookie cutter-like instrument, exactly the same size as the scar itself. Then this tiny punched-out piece of skin pops up to skin level, where it is sewn in place. Later, if there is any irregularity to the skin, a local dermabrasion can be done to smooth it out. This technique is very effective in making these spots look better.

Back Scars

Q: What can be done for the bad acne scars on the back? My doctor uses a cold slush treatment and says that there is very little to do for these types of scars. Is this true?

A: Unfortunately, back scars are the hardest to treat. This is the case where the old cliché, "an ounce of prevention is worth a pound of cure," actually does apply. The scars on the back are so extensive in some kids that almost no therapy helps. I find that the woven, unmedicated acne cleansing pads (like the Buf-Puf), used with slightly drying soaps containing sulfur or benzoyl peroxide, work best to smooth out some small scars, but we really can do practically nothing to help the big sunken scars on the back at this time. Theoretically, Zyderm would work, but small mountains of it might be needed to show significant effect.

You may have noticed from time to time that some acne lesions on the back heal with a nodule or bump above the surface. These are usually reddish at first. They are solid, almost rock-hard. These are called *hypertrophic scars* and are extremely difficult to treat. Sometimes the peeling slush treatment with carbon dioxide, made up by mixing acetone with crushed dry ice, or a spray freezing treatment with liquid nitrogen does help in combination with injections of cortisone right into the scars. Various types of cortisones are used for these shots. (*Note*: These treatments are *only* to be administered by your doctor; they are *never* to be attempted by the patient!) It's these terrifically damaging scars which we hope the new retinoid drugs will help avert in the future.

DERMALERT

The time to take care of acne scarring on the back is before it even appears. When the nodules and bumps begin to form on the back, treat them immediately because they are extremely hard to rehabilitate once the scars have formed.

Special Uses for Zyderm

Q: I am a lymphoma patient who has acne scars. Is Zyderm okay to use on me?

A: In general, yes, so long as you do it with the proper skin tests and in consultation with your dermatologist. Your dermatologist will undoubtedly want to speak to your oncologist or cancer physician to get approval for using Zyderm in your case.

Q: Does the length or size of the scar have any bearing on the effectiveness of the collagen implant treatment?

A: Some of the longest scars have been those following trauma and surgical repair. These scars (some of them on the forehead) are usually quite deep and are filled very well with Zyderm and/ or Zyplast therapy. Deeper defects I have worked on, such as some on the nose after severe injuries, have not filled completely but have been made to look less obvious. Just how Zyderm can be used in surgical defects is illustrated by the following question.

Q: I had plastic surgery on my chin about three years ago. The doctor took out one of my ribs and used it in my chin to cover a defect. Now I have sunken-in places on my chin that I am very self-conscious about. Will Zyderm possibly work here?

A: Some patients have been given as much as twenty milliliters of Zyderm implant material to fill in large defects such as yours. The material, once injected, appears to become a part of the skin, and, as a matter of fact, one's own skin cells *grow into* the material and actually seem to adopt it permanently.

Excluding a monetary factor (because the material is quite expensive), there should be no practical limit to the amount you can have put into a defect, assuming of course the other prerequisites for Zyderm therapy are fulfilled.

Keep in mind that some surgical defects have quite severe scars anchoring the depressed defect to deeper tissues so that the Zyderm implant, which depends upon elevation of the upper layers of the skin, may not be useful in areas of severe restrictive scarring. However, in most cases subsequent treatments are easier because the material tends to soften the preexistent scar.

I would certainly look into Zyderm in your case.

DERMALERT

Zyderm collagen implant can be used to help correct surgical defects and scars as well as acne scars.

Complications of Collagen

Q: What complications can occur in patients receiving Zyderm implants?

A: The main complication, of course, as I have previously mentioned, is allergy to the medicine. While a test injection usually filters out those who are allergic to the medicine, there have been several reports of facial reaction even after negative skin testing. This involved tender bumps lasting several months. Keep in touch with your skin therapist if you have *any* problems whatsoever with your injections.

Other possible complications include (rarely) infection and sun sensitivity in the injection sites. Sun sensitivity causes temporary redness. This can also occasionally occur if a patient drinks alcohol after having the injections. In general, it is wise for Zyderm-injected patients to get minimal sun and avoid alcohol for several days after the injections.

In summary, Zyderm collagen implants have become one of the most useful tools in the dermatologist's arsenal for restoring scarring skin to its normal look. Realize, however, that it does not solve scarring once and for all. It just alters the contour of the skin so that the scarring which is present is less obvious.

In this regard, I remember Maria, a patient who had a special type of acne the French call "acne excoriée des jeunes filles." This means severely picked-at acne of young women. Maria had had a tremendously disturbing youth, and as an expression of this discontent she began picking at the few acne lesions she developed as a teenager.

She became so embroiled with her physical appearance that she would actually try to dig out any small imperfection, such as an acne bump, with her fingernail! The result: large scarred craters in place of acne bumps. When she came to see me her scars were a quarter of an inch deep, and she had become a virtual recluse.

After a negative skin test, we began a program of biweekly Zyderm collagen implant injections which rapidly filled her craters to the point where shadowing from overhead lights was minimal. The craters themselves would never go away, and the pigment she had scratched out probably would never return, but with minor cosmetic adjustments she was able to restore her social functioning to a more normal basis. Now she writes me every few months to let me know how well she is doing with her "new life." It's frankly as close to a cosmetic miracle as I have ever seen!

9

—

Nonacne Problems of
the Young

Beware! All teenage skin problems are not acne! Teens suffer from a tremendous array of skin troubles which have nothing to do with acne even though the teens themselves sometimes think they do. To wit, Harry's story.

Harry, a 19-year-old, complained that he had "a constant battle with acne on strange parts of my body, including areas around my genitals."

"Acne in your groin?" I asked.

"Yep, I've noted little black dots on the skin of my groin and white dots actually on the hairs themselves. My family doctor gave me a prescription for it and told me it was an infection, but it has not gone away. Could it be something else?"

"Well, yes, I believe it could, Harry; indeed it could."

"Well, what then?" Harry asked.

"Lice. Pubic lice. Now, let's take a look and see what's 'bugging' you."

Harry dropped his trousers and revealed a massive infestation with pubic lice. They were crawling everywhere. The nits, or tiny eggs, were adherent to almost every one of his pubic hairs, and even as I watched, Harry could not stop scratching.

"What *are* they?" Harry asked impatiently.

"They're lice, Harry, no question about it," I said. "One of my residency mates had a very apt term for these itchy little critters. He called them 'crotch crickets.'"

I gave Harry a prescription for lindane shampoo, which kills the lice, and told him to treat himself by sudsing up liberally every other day for a week. I also told him to send any sexual contacts he might have had to the Health Department to get checked for the same problem. Later, he told me that he was now very reluctant to call anyone a "louse" again. I've never figured out how his family doctor missed the diagnosis. Maybe he skipped his dermatology course in med school.

Teenagers have a fascinating plethora of changes occurring in their bodies which directly affect the day-to-day comfort of their existence. They're waging not only pitched battles to gain the recognition of their friends and schoolmates, but daily battles with an onslaught of new hormones. And these hormones, as we've seen in Chapter 7, can mark them for life.

Along with teenagers' new hormones come the whole complex series of emotional changes which lead to emotional involvement and sexual contacts, resulting in a host of "new" infectious diseases relating to direct or indirect contact. So, the skin of teenagers must return to war to fight these new invaders.

I am glad that often I get to see a teen early, so that when he or she gets an embarrassing problem later, I'm there, hopefully as a trusted friend as well as a physician, to help them. I had treated one teenager, Mark, months previous for explosive cystic acne, and he now looked terrific. But this trip to the office was for something quite different. He appeared at our front office window and whispered to one of my staff, "May I please talk to Dr. Bark today; I don't have an appointment, and I think it's kind of important."

"Sure, Mark," said my receptionist, sensing a certain determined urgency in his voice, "I'll put you in room 6 and ask Dr. Bark to drop in."

When I arrived, Mark was red-faced and frowning. "Dr. Bark," he said, not meeting my gaze, "I found this on my shoulder this

morning and thought I'd bring it in to you. Can you identify it?"
He held out a small, carefully folded, notebook paper packet.

"I'll sure try, Mark," I said, wondering whether he might be
suffering from delusions of parasitosis. That's a neurotic fear of
things crawling on the skin, though Mark was far from neurotic.
I carefully unfolded the tiny parcel to reveal a single hair with a
single pubic louse, still *alive* and *kicking*, firmly attached to it.

Mark seemed destroyed when I told him he had "caught something from a 'friend.' " It took many minutes of explanation and
a pledge not to inform his parents to calm him down. Finally, I
managed to assure him that he'd survive this embarrassing problem, and so would his girlfriend. As it turned out, she was the
first girl with whom he had had a serious relationship, so it was
a very delicate problem.

In fact, when I think of how many skin problems can affect
teens, it's really a wonder how any of us get to our twenties
without getting some of them!

Lice

Q: I have just been treated for a case of pubic lice but I do
not know where I got it. Could it have been the toilet seat?

A: While *theoretically* you could have picked it up from a toilet
seat, there would have had to have been a fairly direct form of
contact, i.e., you would have had to sit down immediately after
someone else with lice sat there. Lice do not like cold temperatures
and rarely live long if they are deprived of body heat, so that the
toilet seat theory is really difficult to believe with this problem
and with venereal diseases as well.

A much more likely explanation is that you were sexually close
to someone who had the infestation and some of the parasites
crawled onto your skin.

Q: Why do they call pubic lice "crabs"?

A: Under a microscope they look like tiny crustaceans—shell,
claws, and all.

Q: I have used my lindane shampoo to cure my pubic lice
but some of the nits still remain. Am I going to get it back?

A: No. Lindane shampoo kills live lice and incubating eggs of lice (nits) almost immediately. However, you should be careful to wash your underwear in hot soapy water so that you don't get lice back from any nits which might have been deposited in the seams of your clothing. While this is usually a problem only with body lice, it can also be true for pubic lice.

The nits, while still firmly cemented to the hair shaft, are dead if you have used lindane in the prescribed manner.

DERMALERT

Pubic lice almost always results from direct, close contact with another person or sex partner.

Q: My teenage son has gotten head lice and we have treated it, but the nits remain. How can I tell if the nits are flakes of dandruff and how can I remove them?

A: Nits are very easily distinguished from flakes of dandruff by grabbing them with tweezers and trying to slide them up and down the hair shaft. If they do not slide, they are probably nits. If they slide very easily, they are most likely small flakes of dandruff.

Removing these small egg cases from the hairs is extremely difficult. The makers of lindane used to provide a small "nit comb" with their shampoo so that the nits could be combed out after treatment.

One dermatologist suggests a warm vinegar soak as a way to detach these tiny egg shells from the actual hair shaft. It is supposed to work very nicely. It certainly is cheap, and should be harmless if you don't get it in your eyes (where it might sting).

DERMALERT

After a proper lindane treatment for lice, any nits remaining are dead. However, nits should be removed so you can get the child back in school, since nits are the only practical indicator of infestation for the school nurse.

School nurses are quite insistent on the cutaneous health of their children and will almost always refuse to admit children with remaining nits even though they have had the proper therapy prescribed by a dermatologist.

Scabies

Q: My doctor says that my girlfriend and I both have "the itch." What is it, and what can we do about it?

A: The itch is an ancient disease called *scabies* (rhymes with "rabies"). Scabies is an infestation by mites too tiny to be seen with the naked eye. These tiny creatures crawl around just beneath the skin surface, excreting material which causes stupendous itching, especially at nighttime.

The itch has a very famous place in history. It probably lost the Battle of Waterloo for Napoleon. His whole army had the disease and was unable to rest adequately the night before the great battle. As a matter of fact, Napoleon himself had the itchy nuisance for years. Just think of all the paintings of Napoleon you have seen with his hand in his shirt. Historians say he was *scratching* the itch!

Scabies itching, usually worse at night, is most severe between the finger webs and under the armpits and in body folds, the navel area, and very frequently on the head of the penis, a soft spot which mites seem to love.

Scabies can't be definitively diagnosed unless we actually find evidence of the mites' presence. To do this, we scrape off one of the tiny suspicious bumps and apply a small drop or two of potassium hydroxide (KOH). The KOH causes clearing of the skin cells, allowing the protein case of the mite shell to be seen quite clearly under the microscope. Eggs and droppings from the mites can also be seen with great regularity during this test.

DERMALERT

If you're having a lot of itching at nighttime and have bumps between your fingers and your armpits or

around your navel or on your genitalia, you could
have a mite infestation known as scabies.

The incredible itching of scabies at night may result from the
calming of daytime distractions, allowing the itching to surface
into consciousness. However, some investigators feel that the
mites actually move more at nighttime than they do during the
day.

We may not know an answer for why patients itch when they
have scabies, but itch they do! In fact, even after successful treatment of scabies, the itching can last for three or more full weeks.
We call this the "itch of infection." It is probably due to the dead
bodies of mites and the products they leave embedded in the
skin, until the skin has a chance to reproduce itself and shed the
infected areas.

Treatment for scabies is relatively simple, but it has to be done
exactly right. Usually this consists of the application of lindane
lotion to all body skin of every infected family member for twenty-
four hours, once a week, for two to three weeks. While these are
general recommendations, almost every dermatologist has slight
variations in the treatment for his or her own patients. For instance, some dermatologists do not treat infants with lindane. I
don't, because a study some time ago showed toxic effects in
animals who were bathed excessively in the lindane products. In
such cases, crotamiton cream and lotion can be substituted for
lindane, although it is not nearly as effective. It's an even safer,
nonabsorbed insecticide. Crotamiton does, however, have the bonus
of relieving itching as it kills mites, whereas lindane is just a mite
killer.

A scabies patient will do almost anything to relieve the itching.
Will, a painter, had an itchy rash for weeks and discovered his
own "solution" to the problem. Quite early in the course of his
disease he had noticed that he never got the itchy spots on his
hands if he cleansed his hands each day with turpentine or min-
eral spirits. So Will started washing all his itchy areas with turpentine, which quite effectively kept his scabetic infestation down
to a minimum. But then he showed up in my office with severe
turpentine irritation of his skin. It was only coincidentally that I

noticed during the examination of his dry, red, cracked skin that he had some small bumps around his navel and around the head of his penis which looked like classical scabies bumps. Around his navel there were even a few tiny burrows where mites had quite obviously taken up residence. Inspection of his hands, however, revealed no scabies spots there at all. Apparently his "turpentine treatment," while very irritating, was somewhat effective in eradicating the mites.

Tinea Versicolor—Spotted Fungus

Q: My husband started developing whitish spots on his shoulder on our honeymoon when he was still a teenager, and we thought they were water spots from swimming. At first they were only the size of a quarter, but they have now spread over the upper torso. They start out as just dry white patches and then turn whiter than the surrounding skin. He gets very frustrated in the summertime when the lighter color really shows up. He has used many medicines such as Tinactin, but none has ever helped. Is there anything he can use which will get rid of these spots once and for all?

A: Your husband has a fungus infection called *tinea versicolor* (TV). Tinea versicolor is Latin for "many-colored fungus." The name comes from the fact that, during the summertime, the fungus prohibits tanning. To do this it secretes an acid which shuts down the pigment cells in the skin. Occasionally, during the wintertime, they can even look darker than the surrounding skin. As yet, we don't understand exactly why the darker phase occurs. Some scaling accompanies these discolored spots but frequently there are very few symptoms.

The TV fungus is usually caught by direct or indirect contact with someone else who has had it. That is, one can contract the spores of the fungus by using someone else's towel in gym class, by trying on a blouse at a department store after an infected person has done the same and deposited some of the spores, or, of course, by direct skin-to-skin contact.

DERMALERT

Tinea versicolor spots contain thousands of contagious spores. Using another's clothing or towels is
the prime source of contagion.

There appears to be a large factor of individual susceptibility,
however, since not all those who have contact with the fungus
get the disease. Some people obviously have a natural resistance.
Fungus grows very high upon the skin layers so that it is not
really attacked by the body's usually efficient systems of eliminating infections. Even more important, the fungus spores lodge
down inside the hair follicles and can spread back onto the skin
after local treatments have knocked out all the surface fungus.
This fact was amply demonstrated several years ago when electron
microscope pictures of a hair follicle revealed the spores deep
below the surface. It was then that we dermatologists found out
why we had had such little success in treating this stubborn problem.

Since that time, however, we have developed a few new bul-
lets for our treatment gun which can help tremendously. One of
these was the recent discovery that propylene glycol, a common
solvent used to dilute and mix other dermatologic medications,
actually kills this fungus. While this medication is occasionally
slightly irritating, it's extremely safe to use and should be relatively cheap to have mixed up by one's pharmacist on the prescription of a dermatologist. Prior to the advent of propylene
glycol therapy we used a very foul-smelling topical sulfur lotion
called *selenium sulfide* which was applied and left on for a considerable length of time. The stuff was so rotten-smelling that it
would not only obliterate one's fungus but would also blow away
one's relatives if they were anywhere nearby! Thankfully those
days are now passing with the advent of new treatment preparations for this disease. We still use sulfur in a minor way, in
sulfur-containing soaps, which are effective in preventing a recurrence of the fungus for several months after treatment.

Even more recently a new antifungal medicine has been found
to be extremely effective in wiping out this long-term nuisance.
It is ketoconazole (Nizoral), a newly introduced oral antifungal

which treats TV very easily. One only has to take the pills once a day for seven to fourteen days. There have been rare cases of liver irritation with ketoconazole, however, so ask your dermatologist to explain all possible side effects of the drug. He or she may want you to get occasional lab tests to check the status of your liver while you are under treatment for the fungus. Take careful note that although Nizoral is very *effective* in TV, it is *not FDA-approved* for this disease. Many dermatologists will not use it for this indication. *I* do, but only after carefully informing the patient of any possible risks.

DERMALERT

White spots on the skin during the summertime are tinea versicolor fungus infection until proved otherwise. Your doctor can very easily scrape these to make the diagnosis. New medicines allow easier treatment of this annoying disease.

Q: That's all fine and good as an explanation, but will he ever get his tan back?

A: Most assuredly. When the fungus is gone and the pigment suppressor chemical is no longer secreted, the color cells will again turn on their production of normal pigment and the skin will return to its usual shade. It may take some months and a little tan for this to happen, so be patient. If he has any trouble retanning, he should see his dermatologist again for further information and to make sure that he doesn't have either a recurrence of the disease or some other problem associated with lack of pigment.

Teens' Sun Spots

Q: I have white spots on my arms that do not tan even with a lot of sun exposure. They're mostly on the tops of my arms and shoulders. The doctor says it's not fungus. Can you send me more information on this?

A: Assuming you are correct that there is no fungus present in these spots, your most likely diagnosis is *pityriasis alba*. This is Latin for "scaly white spots." This annoying condition is due to dryness and excess sun exposure. It often starts with mild itching and then progresses to whitish flat spots that just won't tan no matter how much sun you get. We also see these more commonly in women on birth control pills.

DERMALERT

Sun, dryness, and the pill can cause annoying white spots on the upper outer arms, called pityriasis alba.

Treatment is far from perfect. It consists usually in moisturizing the spots, sometimes with a cortisone lotion if there is any slightly red component of irritation and scale left. If not, a moisturizing sunscreen such as Coppertone Supershade 15 can be used to solve the dryness and the excess sun exposure problems simultaneously.

The pigment will indeed return; it just takes moisturization and sun avoidance for a while to get the natural-looking skin back.

Keratosis Pilaris—A "Gift" from Parents

Q: I have little, raised, natural skin tone bumps on my upper outer arms and some on the fronts on my legs. My mother had these too. What are they? Do they have anything to do with diabetes or kidney trouble? I have both.

A: These small, spiny, skin-colored bumps around hairs on the backs of the arms are called *keratosis pilaris*. They are a harmless projection of dead skin cells from the hair follicle opening which can be quite a nuisance, having what we call autosomal dominance, i.e., occurring in about 50 percent of the progeny of a patient with the disease.

However simple the condition seems to be, it's one of the most difficult to treat. Most useful has been the polyester nonmedicated sponge (the Buf-Puf) used with slightly acid sulfur soaps for removing the scale. After washing with the sponge and this special soap, you should dry thoroughly, and lavishly apply a moisturizing lotion to soften the hard, scaly bumps. The best lotion for this is a recently developed one called Lac-Hydrin, a prescription moisturizer from the Westwood Company. Other good nonprescription lotions, which you may want to try first, are LactiCare and Complex 15.

DERMALERT

Feel the backs of your arms right now! If the upper backs of your arms have small bumps on them, you've got keratosis pilaris, and each of your children will have a 50 percent chance of getting it.

Mild to moderate sun exposure can also help this condition resolve, but remember that sun exposure causes other damage to your skin, so I would approach sun therapy for keratosis pilaris very moderately, if at all.

To my knowledge, while there are scaly problems of the skin which relate to diabetes and kidney trouble, this is not one of them. Your dermatologist, of course, can give you more information on this. Here is another typical description from the mother of a child with keratosis pilaris.

Q: My 12-year-old daughter has bumps on the backs of her arms above the elbows. They are about the size of pimples but are not characteristic of them. They become red and itching sometimes. Two of her doctors have said that she has thick skin and that the oil is not able to come out. Another doctor, a dermatologist, said this was hereditary but did not tell me what caused them. What can I do for them?

A: Your daughter has an even more extensive and slightly more severe form of keratosis pilaris called *inflammatory keratosis pilaris*. That means the bumps are accompanied by redness and itching. The treatment I mentioned above should help her adequately, but sometimes even antibiotics are necessary to help suppress the inflammation and possible bacterial infection which can result in these red, itchy bumps. In these cases, it's more like treating acne than routine keratosis pilaris.

When your dermatologist said they were hereditary, he actually *did* tell you what caused them. If he was smart enough to tell you what caused the hereditary nature of these, I'm sure he would be flying to Stockholm soon to pick up his Nobel Prize!

Excess Sweating—Completely Treatable

Q: I have tremendous problems with underarm sweating. It's so bad that I can virtually never remove my coat in public because of it. I heard about some "magic medicine" that will stop underarm sweating, and I am in drastic need of that medication. Will you please send some quickly?

A: The problem you're having is an extremely common one called *axillary hyperhidrosis,* or excessive underarm sweating. It's due purely to emotional causes. You can prove this to yourself by looking under your arms if you should wake up in the middle of the night. Virtually everyone is dry at this time. That's because the stresses of the day are no longer with us, and the sweating does not occur.

When I was a resident in dermatology, our training director used to demonstrate this fact by asking us to press a palm against a blackboard. Little, if any, blackness resulted, indicating very little moisture or sweating. Then he would ask us to replace our palms on the blackboard and keep them there while he asked us to perform increasingly more difficult mathematical problems. At the end of two minutes of anxious figuring, there were large wet spots on the blackboard where each of us had secreted volumes of sweat during the stress!

DERMALERT

Stress, and only stress, causes problem underarm sweating.

It is important to remember that there is a type of sweating which is actually needed by the body. This is the insensible, or unnoticed, water we lose during the daytime. This water loss functions to cool the body and to eliminate certain toxins from the system. However, underarm sweating is not a necessary physiologic process. Underarm sweating, and even palmar sweating for that matter, can be shut down very effectively and very safely by using a wonderful medicine called Drysol.

Drysol is a concentrated solution of aluminum chloride in alcohol. It's a prescription medicine which can be obtained only on the advice of and consultation with your dermatologist, because he or she must check your underarms for any skin diseases which would prohibit its use. Also, your dermatologist will teach you how to use it and tell you about the mandatory three steps needed to ensure that you get "clothing-dry underarms." This term, coined by Dr. Walter Shelley when he invented Drysol, indicates that while not all sweating disappears from the underarm, enough disappears so that one never has to worry again about removing layers of clothing in public.

DERMALERT

Stop sweating! Stop using deodorant! You can do it with Drysol, a prescription sweat stopper.

Aluminum chloride slows down and even stops eccrine, or watery, sweating in the underarms. To apply follow the following mandatory steps: (1) Your underarms must be *completely dry*. The medicine cannot be applied immediately after a shower because of residual water in the skin. If necessary, blow-dry the underarms with a hair dryer. (2) After the medicine is applied, put a six- to eight-inch square piece of *plastic wrap* in the armpit to protect your nightclothes from the staining properties of Drysol as well as to hold it on the skin so it will be more effective. (3) Wear a *T-shirt* over your torso during the night to keep the plastic wrap in place.

Drysol *must* be washed off in the morning before clothing is worn. You may think that if leaving it on overnight was effective, possibly leaving it on during the daytime will increase effectiveness, but this is not true. Daytime use is to be avoided because of Drysol's corrosive effects on clothing, and the possible irritation of the tender underarm skin.

The nice thing about Drysol is its infrequency of use. While conventional deodorants are applied daily or more often, Drysol is applied only twice on consecutive nights to start, and only once or twice *per week* thereafter. Fantastic! Sweating stops from the underarms almost instantaneously! This was illustrated quite nicely by a teenage patient of mine named Steve who came in one day wearing a green sport shirt completely soaked with underarm sweat, all the way down to the belt line. He said that he could no longer go on sweating like this and carry on his daily activities.

I made a quick deal with Steve in order to educate more people about Drysol. He agreed to treat only the *right* underarm with the medication for two weeks if we could put him on television to teach people about this marvelous medication.

At the end of the second week, Steve returned for the TV taping with the widest smile I've ever seen. He raised the right arm high in the air revealing a large objectionable patch of sweat! I was quite discouraged until he broke into laughter saying, "Don't worry, Dr. Bark, I switched arms on you!"

Thereupon he raised the left arm and revealed only a tiny, dime-sized drop of moisture! Steve was very proud, and the video tape of his success has helped hundreds of severely sweating patients cope with their problem.

I have treated literally hundreds of other people with various sweating problems, including palm sweating in salespeople, switchboard operators, and others. Occasionally, it's so bad that these patients can cup their hands and sweat a small puddle right before my eyes!

One patient, a gun dealer, was about to give up his business because the sweat from his hands corroded the bluing on gun barrels. After a day or two of Drysol, he went back to work with confidence for the first time in his life. It even works for teenagers whose feet sweat enough to rot their shoes.

For those who need it, Drysol certainly passes the "Callaway" test. The Callaway test was originated by Dr. J. Lamar Callaway from the Duke University Department of Dermatology, who stated that a truly effective medicine is the one for which the patient brings back an empty bottle and says, "Doctor, I've got to have some more of *this* stuff!" In other words, a medicine that works!

Body Odor

Q: You mentioned a technique for stopping perspiration, but my 15-year-old daughter has a problem with underarm *odor*. She showers daily and uses a deodorant and antiperspirant, but when she gets home from school, she has terrible underarm odor. She has been using deodorants since she was about 3 years old! What can we do?

A: The Drysol technique for stopping perspiration may indeed help your daughter, but it's more important to know what causes the odor from underarms so that you can prevent it. There are generally two types of bacteria on the human skin. The first are gram-positive bacteria, which normally live on the skin. But some, like staph, can sometimes infect the skin and cause problems, the chief of which is body odor. The second type is the gram-negative type. These usually originate in the bowel areas and are normally on the skin only in very small numbers.

Deodorants fight body odor by killing off the more common gram-positive bacteria. This allows the less common gram-negative bacteria to multiply in the underarms. That's good, because they don't smell. But Drysol is an *antiperspirant* which actually stops sweating. In most cases Drysol will solve this problem by decreasing wetness, but in some, the malodorous secretions still continue even after Drysol therapy.

A very simple therapy for underarm odor, therefore, is to use a topical antibiotic which cuts down on the numbers of gram-positive bacteria. While most "deodorant soaps" have antibacterial properties, they are not strong enough for difficult cases like your daughter's. In such situations, topical antibiotics such as neomycin can help amazingly. Ask your dermatologist about this and other antibiotics such as topical cleocin, erythromycin, and garamycin. There is really no need for her to have this problem.

DERMALERT

Underarm *sweating* can be shut down with Drysol. In the case of underarm *odor*, topical antibiotics can stop the problem most efficiently.

Failure to Sweat

Q: My daughter has very, very dry skin and does *not* perspire. We were watching a parade in the sun one day and she nearly passed out in what was not excessive heat for a normal person. She is 32 years old now and I wonder if something can be done to help her. Last year she took aerobic dancing and her pulse soared to over 200!

A: Your daughter appears to have complete or nearly complete absence of sweat glands, a disorder called *congenital anhidrotic ectodermal defect*. This condition leaves the victim without one of the body's most important cooling mechanisms, that of evaporative sweating. Without this major air-conditioning device, tolerance for heat is almost nil. These people can have heat strokes in even mildly elevated temperatures.

It's vital for your daughter to visit a dermatologist skilled in the evaluation of this condition, so that the presence or absence of sweat glands and their normal function can be documented. If indeed she has congenital anhidrotic ectodermal defect, then she will need to avoid hot environments at all costs. As yet, we have no other therapy for the condition.

Sunlamps

One other topic that affects teenagers should be included in this chapter—sunlamps. While we'll be discussing sunlamps more thoroughly in Chapter 17, I must take this opportunity to warn teens that there are good documented cases of sun "therapy" causing permanent damage to the skin of the face. These can include bad attacks of sun-induced acne.

I try to warn people about the adverse effects of sunlight and sunlamps whenever I get the chance, and I couldn't risk leaving a section written for teenagers without mentioning sun damage.

A final note: If you're a teen with a problem, don't be afraid to talk to your doctor about it. It won't be the first time he or she has heard about the problem, or the first time he or she has treated it in a teen. While there are many people one should not trust these days, your doctor is one you *can* trust.

10

Hair—Either Famine or Feast

Chrome dome, baldy, skin head. We've all heard these terrible terms poking fun at men who have lost all or part of their hair. The use of such terms shows the almost universal importance of hair in our society as an indicator of virtually hundreds of different personality traits.

For instance, here are the results of a recent study published in the *St. Louis Globe Democrat*: Seventy-five percent of bald or balding executives surveyed agreed that their social life was affected by their hair loss. Ninety percent thought there was not enough research to find a cure, and a whopping seventy-one percent thought bald men were not as well accepted by society as those with hair.

Billions of dollars are spent on male and female hair care in our society each year. Hair is a vital component in the interaction between men and women. Whenever I have spoken before large groups, I've been deluged with hair questions. Many of the questions in this chapter were derived from those. This chapter covers many different types of hair loss in some detail to tell the whole story of what we know and don't know about their causes and treatment. We'll discuss several experimental forms of treatment for hair loss. You should *know* about these treatments even if they're not yet FDA-approved or widely available in your area; so if they prove to greatly help hair loss, you'll already be familiar with them.

Beyond the investigational measures to solve hair loss, you should know about proper everyday hair care, especially if you're *losing* hair. And there are so many quacks and charlatans waiting to get their hands upon your balding head; you must know how to avoid *their* clutches above all! So hang on to your hair as we discuss the many questions about hair loss and hair care.

Male Pattern Baldness

Q: I am 26 years old and have been losing my hair for about six years! I have not lost all of my hair but could probably get into the I-hate-it-when-the-wind-blows club with no trouble. Why me?

A: Ever since Hippocrates treated baldness with a sludge of opium, rose petals, and unripe olives, the treatment of baldness has been a major human concern. Many men feel that if they don't have hair, life is just not worth living. Our questioner is one of those I call "wrappers." A wrapper lets one long scalp lock grow out of the horseshoe area of remaining hair, so that he can wrap it around and around and around, spray it with hairspray or some other kind of glue, and partially cover his bald pate. I once knew a guy like this who would go out jogging in the wind, and at the end of a single block would look like a shaved Cossack with a single, long, flowing scalplock!

Other men calmly allow their baldness to progress and, I think, more or less feel it is a sign of virility more than anything else. It's hard to predict the way people will react to a problem which so obviously affects the way they greet the world and the way it greets them. But why do we lose hair? What can be done to hang on to what we have?

Male pattern baldness is called *androgenetic alopecia* (AGA). The term "androgenetic" tells a lot about the origin and expression of the condition. First of all, it is necessary to have the primary genetic material in order to go bald. That is, if you don't have the hair loss genes, you don't lose hair.

The genes, of course, are passed down through families by the male *and* the female members. It's a common fallacy that only the males in the family carry the gene, and that if your father had a full head of hair, you will automatically have one. But the gene does indeed pass on either side of the family; so it is necessary to search the family tree on *both* sides to find the link to the member with hair loss.

DERMALERT

Baldness is a genetic condition. The gene is passed down by both male *and* female members.

Besides the gene for baldness, it's also necessary to have the androgenic or male hormones required to activate the baldness gene. The situation may be likened to a lawnmower in a yard full of grass. The grass cannot be cut (baldness) without three prerequisites. First, the lawnmower (the gene) has to be there. Second, gasoline (the androgenic hormone) has to be put in the lawnmower. Last, the engine cord must be pulled (age) to start the lawnmower.

The chief hormone I mentioned is called dihydrotestosterone (DHT). DHT is a very potent cause of "miniaturization" of the male hair follicle. Miniaturization? Yes, I mean exactly that; bald men are not bald at all. Their long, black, adult "terminal" hairs have just evolved into baby-fine "vellus" hairs which are invisible, or nearly so, to the naked eye.

But the follicles themselves, which are the hair-producing units, are still intact. This leaves hope for future medicines which may be used to turn on those miniaturized hair follicles. We shall talk more about this later when we talk about treatment for male pattern loss.

Age is the final trigger for the onset of baldness. One of the many mysteries of baldness is why a young man of 19 who has the same hormones and genes that he will have at 45 often does not lose hair at the former age but will have lost perhaps much of it at the latter.

Dr. Norman Orentreich, the great hair expert and inventor of the hair transplant, likes to relate a story about identical twins, one of whom was castrated before puberty because of a testicular disease. His brother lost hair, but the castrated twin did not. At about age 40 he received a series of shots containing male hormone. Six months later he was precisely as bald as his twin. He had needed the hormonal "key" to activate his hair loss.

Vitamins

Q: I'm convinced that my hair thinning on the top of my head is due to a vitamin deficiency, because I'm the world's most avid junk food eater. Which vitamins do I really need to get my hair to return?

A: Vitamin deficiency does not cause hair loss except in the most dire circumstances. Many starving children of Bangladesh began to lose their hair which also underwent color changes before the children died from malnutrition. It's nearly impossible to find that type of malnutrition on this continent. Of course, there are certain disease states, such as cancer and alcoholism, in which malnutrition can be this severe, but these are by far the exceptions. Don't waste your money on vitamin therapies. This includes all the special "hair vitamins" advertised in the lay press.

DERMALERT

Don't believe vitamin theories about hair loss. To do so is to chase wild geese for years on end, a very costly pursuit!

Q: Does wheat germ shampoo have a tendency to cause hair loss because of the wheat germ content?

A: I can only tell you that several world-famous hair experts have advised us dermatologists to have our patients avoid wheat germ in any form. I used a wheat germ shampoo myself for a year or two, because I liked its fragrance, but I too gave it up when I heard that wheat germ might possibly encourage hair loss.

The oil in wheat germ contains a male hormone-like substance which resembles that which causes AGA. Certainly it would be wise to avoid any possible source of such substances.

Q: I saw an ad in a men's magazine with a questionnaire which I was supposed to fill out and send in, so they could determine how to help me with my hair loss. I sent it in with my check, but I didn't get anything back! Why don't you warn people about this?

A: Consider yourself warned. It's always been amazing to me how quick people are to fire off a check to a charlatan who has never seen them before. And often how reluctant they can be to visit a dermatologist with the necessary experience to *properly* evaluate their hair loss.

Q: I saw an ad in a magazine for a "hair restorer." Do they work? Mine surely didn't!

A: A patient once remarked in frustration, "If topical hair restorers worked, you'd have hairy *fingers* from applying them!"

While this is an exaggeration, you are one of millions of balding males who are victimized by baldness and hair growth quackery each year. Most often the photographs and advertisements in men's magazines (and women's magazines, for that matter) are retouched photographs showing hair regrowth which cannot possibly occur with these methods. The other trick these charlatans use is to show a type of hair loss called *alopecia areata* in which the hair regrows in almost *everyone* within six months. They pick a person with this disease in a spot where a person might ordinarily have male pattern hair loss, claim it *is* male pattern hair loss, and then show its "rapid regrowth."

Of course, all of these products are worthless. There is not a certified agent currently available which will regrow hair in a person who has lost it due to androgenetic alopecia. However, transplants can work wonders for the proper candidates.

Transplants

Q: I'm desperate. Tell me everything you know about hair transplants.

A: In AGA, hair can often be replaced by moving some of your hair. The transplant surgeon takes out small plugs of bald skin on the crown and replaces them with slightly larger plugs of good hair-bearing skin from the donor sites, usually at the sides of the scalp. (No, if you want curly hair, they will *not* take the donor plugs from your armpits!)

The surgery is usually bloody and very expensive. It can involve scarring, infection, and even rejection of the transplanted plugs. It cannot be overemphasized that you must have this done by a very qualified dermatologic surgeon or plastic surgeon. You must discuss predicted final results, progressive balding requiring further transplants, and all the complications involved.

Sometimes your plastic surgeon may want to do a "scalp reduction" operation before starting your transplant. In this procedure, some of the bald skin is cut away first, leaving a much smaller area to transplant later.

Q: Why do transplant plugs continue to grow hair when they are put in a scalp which has lost its regular hair?

A: There is some genetic component of remaining hairy scalp areas that keeps hairs growing even when transplanted to a new location. We don't know exactly what this factor is yet, but we do know that those hairs grow well, even when the surrounding skin has no obvious terminal hair growth.

Q: Will my transplanted hairs fall out when I lose all my hair?

A: Yes. The transplanted hairs will keep growing until exactly the same time that the donor areas begin to go bald. Luckily most people retain the hairs around the edge of the scalp for a considerably longer time. Therefore, most hair transplantees will not have to worry about this problem, since their plugs are taken from areas which have good hair growth and probably will keep it.

Headgear Hair Loss

Q: My dad warns me about wearing my football helmet because he says that when he played football that's what caused *his*
hair loss. Am I going to have to give up my favorite sport?

A: Absolutely not! The number of old wives' tales (old husbands' tales in this case) concerning a cause for baldness exceed
even the number of patients who are balding. Circulation has
very little to do with hair loss. It's not hard to prove this if one
sees the tremendous bleeding which can occur with scalp lacer-
ations. The scalp actually has the best circulation of any skin on
the human body.

Hair Analysis

Q: I go to a holistic doctor who has advised me to have a
hair analysis done; it's quite expensive and I'd like you to let me
know if it will help or not. I don't have any diseases that I know
of.

A: This extremely sensitive technique for analyzing the
chemicals of the hair has been called nearly valueless by some of
the world's leading hair experts. *Of course* it can tell you what's
in your hair. The problem is that it also tells you what's *on* your
hair! In other words we have so many pollutants, chemicals, and
other matter in the air around us, that these sensitive tests can
be completely thrown off by the substances in the air around your
hair. You could, for instance, live in downtown New York City
and have a completely different hair analysis than your identical
twin who lives uptown. Also, the presence of cigarette smoke
and other pollutants in our environment as well as hair creams,
shampoos, and sprays makes these tests essentially useless. Only
in a rare genetic malformation of the hair, with an *absence* of certain
amino acids, can these tests be of any help.

Real hair experts do not perform many hair analyses. But the
self-styled hair "experts" do, and they'll be very willing to sell
you one of these tests in order to further the current holistic hype.

Consult a real hair expert, your dermatologist, who has studied hair, its growth pattern, its makeup, and its diseases for *years.* You'll get straight information that you can really use.

Massages

Q: My wife is trying to talk me into getting a series of massages to solve my hair loss problem. Will this help?

A: Not in the least! The scalp circulation is already excellent, as I've mentioned, and massaging it will do nothing to help it further.

Minoxidil—A New Light for Hair Loss

Q: We've heard you talk about a new medicine for growing hair. My husband would love to try it, even though it's not perfected yet. He has tried everything, even dog medicine (it grew hair on the dog but not on my husband)! Please tell us about it.

A: The medicine I talked about, and which has inspired virtually hundreds of inquiries, is minoxidil. This potent medication is used internally in very difficult cases of hypertension (high blood pressure), and was discovered to cause hair growth in areas which are not ordinarily covered with it. The medicine, when taken orally, is a very potent stimulator of hair growth, especially on the faces of females where, of course, it's usually neither found nor desired.

This discovery prompted the dermatologic community and the Upjohn Company, makers of the drug, to consider using this medication in the treatment of male pattern hair loss. But since there are many side effects to the medication, it was necessary to plan an extraordinarily careful study to show any possible effectiveness of, and reaction to, the medicine. These studies are now in progress at several centers around the country.

Preliminary results indicate that minoxidil (which will be called Regaine when and if the FDA approves it for prescription use by dermatologists) does in fact produce noticeable regrowth of hair in about 30 percent of men under 40. In another 30 percent or so, the drug seems to help maintain the hair that the patient has currently. The remaining 30 to 40 percent of men have little or no regrowth.

It also seems important to start the medication as soon as possible after hair loss begins. The good news, again from the preliminary reports, is that there are very few, if any, complications yet reported with the medication.

The costs? I've heard estimates for one month's therapy ranging from $40 to $125! Yep, that's expensive, but we all know men who would consider hair replacement well worth that amount.

DERMALERT

New medicines which may even *reverse* baldness are currently under investigation.

Q: How does topical minoxidil work?
A: Minoxidil is a very potent vasodilator. This means that it opens up blood vessels quite widely and, through this mechanism, appears to reduce blood pressure when taken internally. It may be, therefore, that the effect of hair regrowth is produced by some action upon the blood vessels surrounding hairs. We know, however, that circulation is not the reason for baldness. Over thirty years of experience with hair transplants shows us that the donor site hairs will definitely live in areas of balding, so the circulation is fine in balding areas.

Thus there must be something else to the action of minoxidil that we do not yet understand. Regardless, it will be several years before the studies are completed, and judging from past results with medications used in baldness, I would not expect miracles before the final results of the studies are known.

Cyproterone

Q: I would like to know about the use of a steroid called *cyproterone* in male pattern baldness.
A: Cyproterone is a potent antiandrogen which has been under

study in Europe for some time. It works well for females but only when taken internally. The stuff is apparently not active when applied topically.

We are unable to use it in males because, taken internally, this very potent antiandrogen would knock out all the effects of male hormones, which men are unwilling to give up for the sake of saving their hair. These include loss of sexual potency and the development of secondary female sex characteristics such as enlarged breasts. The company making the drug (which, incidentally, is not available in this country) is trying to develop a topically active form of it, but we have no information other than to say that in the future such a drug may be a possibility. The antiandrogen activity of this drug would have to be limited to the skin and not affect the total body when absorbed through the skin. This may prevent cyproterone from ever being used with men.

Progesterone

Q: I've heard that some men are having progesterone injected into the scalp to hang on to whatever hair they've got. Will this help me?

A: To understand how progesterone might work, it is necessary to look much closer at the cells involved in hair loss. If the cells of the hair follicle are genetically predisposed to baldness, they are very sensitive to androgens. You can think of these cells as having tiny piers sticking out from them to which androgens, or male hormones, attach. When this happens, the message brought in by the androgens (a message which tells the cells to miniaturize the hair) is unloaded at the pier and taken into the cell. Progesterone, on the other hand, can be compared to an *empty* barge which pulls into the pier, preventing the attachment of the "boat load of androgen." It is hoped that the barge (progesterone) will keep out the androgen and encourage the hair to be maintained. Some dermatologists inject progesterone into the scalp on a monthly basis to try to *maintain* the hair a man has left.

Personally, I prefer to try minoxidil, which many of us pre-scribe already. We have pharmacists mix it up in solution form for application to the scalp. Be aware, however, that the FDA has issued a caution advising against this practice. If you use minox-idil, please be aware that there may be side effects that are as yet undiscovered.

Daily Washing Helps!

Q: Is there anything else that can help me slow my hair loss?

A: Yes, indeed! It appears that the hormone DHT is secreted in the oil of the sebaceous (or oil) gland which attaches to every hair follicle in the scalp. Thus, the hormone lies upon the surface skin and is therefore reabsorbed through the skin, thereby causing *further loss* when it reaches the hair follicle again. The "circulation" of this potent hair loss-causing hormone can be intercepted through a very simple technique—daily washing! That's right, daily wash-ing can slow down male pattern hair loss! Use an excellent oil-removing shampoo such as X-seb, X-seb-T, Dermalab X5, Der-malab X5T, or Ionil T Plus on a daily basis. The hair should be lathered twice in order to ensure oil removal.

"Age Thinning"

Q: What can help my thinning hair? As a 71-year-old lady, I need all I can hang on to!

A: The hair loss which occurs in females in middle age and later is also a type of pattern hair loss. Sometimes it can occur in the male pattern on the crown, but more often it occurs along the lateral or side areas of the scalp, near the temples, and involves the receding hairline.

Females, of course, have a hormonal situation which resembles that of males, but it occurs later in life. The key is that at meno-pause the ovaries go into an inactive state and stop producing estrogen.

DERMALERT

Women lose hair through an androgenetic mechanism also. This usually happens after menopause, when they lose the protective influence of their natural estrogen.

Work has been done for women with a compound called *estradiol*. This compound in an alcoholic base is a metabolic breakdown product of estrogen and seems to tie up at the little "docks" where androgen normally attaches. It can be applied to the scalp topically after menopause and may indeed slow or halt female pattern loss. It needs to be applied daily but can be effective in helping slow the loss. Minoxidil is under investigation for this type of loss, too.

Q: I'm losing twenty or thirty hairs *a day*! What could be wrong?

A: Nothing! It's been very adequately calculated that hair fall can consist of 100 or 125 hairs a day and still be normal. You essentially have no problem. This question is often brought up in my office and it usually results because a person has just *noticed* their normal hair loss and is now watching for it more.

DERMALERT

Hair loss of 100 to 125 hairs a day is perfectly normal.

Thin Hair in Children

Q: My granddaughter has very thin hair. In fact, she is 2½ years old and does not have enough hair to even put a barrette in. My question is whether or not she is lacking something in her diet. Should she be taking some special vitamin?

A: The fact that she doesn't have enough hair to put a barrette in may be because she has worn them in the past. Barrettes are an occasional cause of a problem we call *traction alopecia*. In this condition, the hair loss is due to chronic, slow pulling on the hair. Barrettes can do this!

As I've said previously, vitamins are not likely to be the problem unless she's on a starvation diet. I've seen several patients who have participated in weight loss programs (sometimes even those overseen by physicians) that have caused drastic amounts of hair loss.

The larger question for your granddaughter is, however, does she have a structural defect in her hair? There are several genetic conditions in which the hairs do not form correctly, having either weak spots or holes within the shaft, causing easy breakage. One of these peculiar diseases is called *trichorrhexis nodosa*. It is characterized by extremely frayed weak spots in the hair shafts which, under the microscope, look like two broomsticks shoved together. It's very easy to snap off the hairs at these weak spots. Your dermatologist can pull a few hairs and spot these strange disorders very quickly.

Treatment for this problem amounts to keeping a short hair style, and avoiding manipulation whenever possible. Avoiding combing when wet will also reduce stresses on hair, and hair conditioners smooth the combing process.

Most people who have thin hair have a family tendency toward it and nothing can be done for this. As you can see, it's important to obtain the correct advice about how to manage easily damaged hair. Perhaps the following question will help.

Proper Hair Care

Q: My hair comes out a lot when I brush or comb it, and after I wash it, I get a lot of breakage. What can I do about this?

A: First of all, stop mishandling your hair! Go get your hairbrush right now, okay? Now, take it out to the nearest lake and give it the strongest throw you can toward the center of the lake! Then only the fish will be damaged by it if they try to brush their scales with it! All kidding aside, hairbrushes are murder on your hair. The tension applied by the conventional hairbrush is so great that it can split, rip, and crack even the strongest of hair shafts.

Worse yet, your question implies that you are combing it when it's *wet*. Stop that! A Caucasian who combs the hair wet exerts terrific forces upon it. Let it get at least partially dry before starting to comb. And be sure to use a wide-toothed comb!

The situation with blacks is the opposite. Blacks with curly hair should start combing gently with a wide-toothed comb when the hair *is* wet. The natural curliness allows it to spring apart so that the water acts more as a separator of the hair shafts and makes combing easier.

Your hair shafts are inherently tough. They should withstand most forces in your daily life without having much splitting, fraying or breakage. The old axiom, "Brush 100 strokes every day," is as ridiculous as a mechanic who tells you to drive your car 100 miles per hour eight hours per day in order to keep your tires in good shape! This folklore started when there were no conditioning shampoos or rinses. It was necessary then to comb out the natural scalp oil and spread it onto the hairs by frequent brushing. With today's modern shampoos and conditioners, this is no longer even the slightest problem.

And that's the take-home message: use a conditioner. These agents drastically reduce the tension exerted on hairs by combing after washing. They coat and smooth the hairs with protein and other chemicals to keep them from tangling. Then combs glide across hairs smoothly, without exerting much force.

Something should be said about the frequency of your shampooing. Shampooing up to once a day does *not* cause increased hair loss or fracturing.

Hair dryers and manipulation are frequent causes of hair loss. I really don't mind hair dryers if they're used properly. By this I mean that a dryer should be used *without* an *attached* comb or brush. Did you ever think about how much your dryer weighs, and how much more force it exerts than using just a simple wide-toothed comb? It's considerable! So use a blow dryer if you wish, preferably on the warm instead of the hot setting, and take off the attached comb or brush.

Of course, hot combs, hot rollers, and hot dryers are incredibly destructive to your hair. A hot comb can induce enough damage to completely fracture hairs, especially along the temple areas, where they're used most often.

Pregnancy and Hair Loss

Q: My husband and I just had our third healthy baby in November, and then in January, I lost a significant amount of hair. Is there anything I can do?

A: There is only one type of hair loss dermatologists enjoy seeing in their offices, and yours is that type! It is called "resting phase loss," or *telogen effluvium.* In order to understand this, it's necessary to know a bit about the way hairs grow normally.

The scalp hair cycle has three different stages. The first of these is the time of active growth called the *anagen* phase. This is the longest phase and can last several years for scalp hairs. During this time healthy follicles are taking in normal amounts of body nutrients and the cells of the follicle are cranking out large amounts of keratin, the special hair protein which makes up the shaft. It's really a time of remarkable activity in the microscopic factory we know as the hair follicle. But it can only last so long.

After four to seven years in most people, the scalp hairs cycle into a regression or involution stage called the *catagen* phase. During this stage, which lasts only a matter of days, the hair follicle shrivels at the end, signifying that its long anagen growth cycle is over. Growth stops quite abruptly now.

Following the catagen phase, the hair develops a bulbous enlargement at the end and is called a *club hair.* The club hair slowly splits off from the follicle. This *telogen hair,* as it's called, remains above the shriveled-up follicle for another month or two, until it is naturally sloughed out by pulling stresses on the outside hair such as combing and wind.

Resting hairs are the ones which come out when you pinch a bunch of hairs and very gently pull away from the scalp. The two or three hairs you obtain in this way were destined to fall out anyway, so don't think you've lost those hairs permanently. They're just cycling through their last phase before starting the new growth cycle.

After several months, telogen phase follicles cycle again into the growth, or anagen, phase.

The trick is understanding the type of hair loss you're having. Over 85 percent of the 100,000 hairs on your scalp are in the active growing phase during most of your life. Only a small amount—some 10 percent or so—are in the resting phase at any one time. In pregnancy, hormonal influences for growth apply not only to the enlarging fetus but also to a woman's own hair. It's locked into the anagen growth phase! This means that pregnant women often have long, luxurious locks growing by leaps and bounds. After delivery, however, the hormones normalize again and the hairs which were locked into the growth phase cycle simultaneously into the catagen and telogen phases. This means that a tremendous number of hairs are ready to fall out after their long stimulus to growth. And they *do!* Some women lose as much as *30 to 40 percent* of their hairs during this period.

DERMALERT

Fully 85 percent of a person's 100,000 hairs are in the active growth cycle at any one time.

Here's the key. The hairs slowly regain their asynchronous cycling nature, which means that they begin to cycle independently of one another again. This means that almost every woman will get her hair back beautifully, as it was prior to her pregnancy, in just a few months. I know this is a little hard to believe when you're seeing handfuls of hair fall out after the birth of your baby, but it is true, and your dermatologist will reassure you of this fact. Stop worrying!

Hair Loss on the Pill

Q: I stopped taking birth control pills several months ago but my hair is falling out like my sister's after she had a baby. I have *never* been pregnant! Will I get my hair back too?

A: Most definitely! The pill simulates the hormonal situation of pregnancy, and therefore locks hairs into growth in most women. While it is true that some women *lose* hair from the pill, most actually have increased hair growth.

DERMALERT

Hair loss after having a baby or stopping the birth control pill will almost always reverse itself.

Q: I had a baby girl four years ago and my usually thick healthy hair began falling out in huge clumps four months after she was born. I think I probably lost a third or more of it! It has not grown back in *four years.* Is there any hormone or other solution to this problem, or must I live with thin hair for the rest of my life?

A: The hair loss you had after you delivered was certainly consistent with telogen effluvium. However, there may have been more than just that going on. Talk with your dermatologist or gynecologist about this. There are many endocrine gland problems which can cause hair loss. Certainly your dermatologist will want to know your menstrual history since the time of your delivery. He or she also will want to test you for the presence or absence of normal hormonal function in your ovaries, adrenals, and pituitary. All these glands are important in determining how much hair a woman has.

Although four years is a long time to expect regrowth, some of your hair indeed may grow back if you have a gland problem which can be solved. I encourage you to get this checked out.

Drugs

Q: I am on Lanoxin to strengthen my heart and propranolol for high blood pressure. Recently I started having thinning of my hair, and I wondered if it's possibly caused by the Inderal?

A: Propranolol may have caused thinning of your hair. Several cases have been reported, and you should ask the physician prescribing it to consider this as a cause for your hair loss. Your physician may want to substitute another medication for a period of several months to see if your hair regrows. This process of elimination is often the only way to ascertain the real cause of hair loss.

Scalp Acne

Q: I have acnelike bumps all through my scalp, and some of them have small pus pockets in them. Am I going to lose my hair because of this?

A: It's probable you will lose some hair. There are many causes of inflammation around hairs which can cause hair loss. Inflammation of the follicle (hair-making unit) is frequently caused by fungal and bacterial infection. The one you seem to have is called *bacterial folliculitis*. The control of bacterial folliculitis on the scalp is very difficult. You may need to be seeing a dermatologist regularly, but it's better than losing one hair with each of the bumps you get. Antibiotics and special treatment shampoos can usually control folliculitis quite nicely.

Alopecia Areata

Q: I have been plagued with bald spots appearing from time to time on my head. My beautician says it is called *alopecia* and it's caused by nerves. The hair comes in after a time but then the baldness reappears in a different spot. At the present time I have two spots in the hairline on the neck. A relative who is a pharmacist has gotten me a special shampoo, which she says should help the hair come in and strengthen it also. What do you think?

A: It sounds like you have *alopecia areata* (AA), which means "area baldness." These well-delineated or "punched out" spots fall out in a matter of days for reasons which are incompletely understood. Studies of this disease indicate that it may be a type of autoimmune reaction; that is, the body is reacting defensively to its own skin and hair follicles, quite an unusual and rare situation.

As I've mentioned before, alopecia areata, or area baldness, is the kind of hair loss for which charlatans and hair treatment quacks used to demonstrate, in their "magnificent photographs," the apparently magical regrowth due to their usually harmless and always ineffective potions. But with this kind of loss the hair regrows on its own within six months. The natural pattern of AA is therefore one of healing.

Unfortunately, sometimes, as in your case, the disease lasts longer and gets much worse. A single spot will regrow hair, and new spots will erupt elsewhere.

The old-timers in dermatology used to think that AA was always related to emotions or a nervous condition, but that's hogwash. Although there are some well documented cases of alopecia areata resulting from severe psychic trauma and mental upset, these are by far the exception rather than the rule. This is another case where physicians tend to attribute a disease entity to an emotional cause when the real physiologic basis for the problem is unknown.

Treatment of alopecia areata is quite varied and depends upon the type you have. With isolated spots, it may be easy to get your hair back by having your dermatologist inject the spots with a dilute triamcinolone solution. This cortisone medication stays inside the skin, working to restore the hair for three to four weeks. In some cases, the injection functions as a permanent "cure," in that the hair does not fall out again. In other cases, it does fall out again, and new spots may even develop.

A slight hazard with the injection is that it can sometimes result in thinning of the skin and an irregular surface contour lasting for some months. However, the skin almost always returns to its original contour.

Other treatments work by inducing irritation on the scalp. One of the older remedies used by dermatologists is croton oil, a strong primary irritant that induces redness, inflammation, and soreness in the scalp. When this occurs, AA will sometimes resolve. Because of the extensive irritation, however, use of croton oil has been largely abandoned.

Other medications causing a healing irritation include anthralin, a plant derivative usually used in psoriasis to slow down the turnover of the epidermis. In alopecia areata it is used to cause irritation of the type that croton oil causes, but in a much more controlled fashion. It is not completely effective, though a significant percentage of patients *will* regrow their hair. Here again the irritation is the most important factor. If your scalp doesn't get irritated, you will not regrow hair. Even if it does get irritated, the regrowth process can take many months.

Recently, immunotherapy for alopecia areata has been developed. This investigational treatment involves the application of a chemical to which one can really get allergic, such as DNCB (dinitrochlorobenzene), or poison ivy resin. Such a chemical is first applied several times to the skin in order to induce allergy, and then a lower concentration is applied to the scalp. Redness, swelling, and sometimes even blisters result. The goal is to cause a little mild redness and keep it there chronically.

The principle appears to be nearly the same as the "primary irritation" produced by croton oil and anthralin. Researchers think that the effectiveness of immunotherapy depends upon the calling up of the body's own lymphocytes, or defense cells, which actually suppress the allergy. It seems to be a case of one immune or allergic reaction canceling out the disease. It's a miserably itchy treatment, but sometimes works to regrow hair.

In short, we don't know exactly how this all comes about, but research is under way to get the safest possible allergen that causes the least reaction and still grows hair. Over the next few years we should see great advances in this particular form of therapy for AA.

Another treatment for AA is called PUVA. While we'll discuss this new development mainly in regard to psoriasis in Chapter 16, you should know that, in some AA patients, PUVA has restored hair *dramatically*.

The PUVA treatment involves taking an oral medicine called Oxsoralen, which makes the skin tremendously sensitive to the sun. In fact, it binds to the skin cell DNA (the actual molecules which control how the skin grows), causing damage to cell growth mechanisms. Two hours after the medicine is taken, the patient is exposed to long-wave ultraviolet light (UVA). PUVA is thus named from the *P*soralen and the *UVA*.

If you want to know more about PUVA and its use in AA, talk to a dermatologist. There are complications with this therapy which you need to understand before undertaking it. Recently, many of these complications have been circumvented by the initiation of treatment with topically applied psoralens, instead of the internally taken type.

Lastly, with regard to alopecia areata, there is a drug on the horizon which we discussed earlier in the section on male pattern loss: minoxidil, a medicine commonly used to treat hypertension.

Topical minoxidil works to regrow hair in some alopecia areata patients. Dr. Virginia Weiss at the University of Illinois is currently doing a study, in cooperation with Dr. Vera Price at Stanford, in which this medicine is being looked at very carefully in regard to use with patients such as the one described in the following question. (Refer to the section on minoxidil for a more detailed discussion.)

Q: My 12-year-old son is almost completely bald with alopecia areata. We have tried various creams, vitamins, and ointments, as well as cortisone injections. These have made it regrow for a short time, but then it falls out again. We live in constant fear that his hairpiece (which he wears to school) will fall off in front of people. Please tell me if there is any way that this can be helped.

A: Your son has a particularly difficult condition. In cases such as his, we have had extreme trouble getting the hair back safely. While it is almost always possible to get these kids' hair to regrow with high to moderate doses of cortisone taken internally, this medication itself has extensive side effects when taken on a long-term basis. Therefore, no one relishes the prospect of putting a child on an internal cortisone medication that he or she might have to stay on for years.

I do not approach internal cortisone treatment lightly, and neither should you. When injected locally into the spots of AA it's certainly safe, and very little absorption occurs to change other body systems. However, when cortisone is given internally in fairly high doses, as needed to regrow his hair, such complications as salt and fluid retention, bone reabsorption, cataracts, ulcers, and psychosis can—and have—occurred.

In your son's case, the most logical thing to do would be to take him to one of the larger medical centers in which some of the newer investigative therapies I have described, such as DNCB and PUVA, are being used.

For now, however, your choice of a hairpiece to help him live a normal life is the wisest course. In most cases of extensive AA, called *alopecia totalis*, almost all the hair has gone from the head area. With some children, every hair on the body falls out, a condition called *alopecia universalis*. These two conditions are occasionally associated with internal problems, such as anemias and thyroid difficulties, so your physician will probably want to check your son for any possible abnormalities.

In the meantime, realize that your son is not the only one with this condition. There are hundreds of patients like your son who are struggling every day with alopecia areata. Recently, the National Alopecia Areata Foundation (NAAF) has been formed to help such victims. You may write to them at:

The National Alopecia Areata Foundation
168 Buchanan Street
Sausalito, California 94965

The NAAF will be more than glad to keep you posted on new developments in treatment, as well as offer advice on ways you and your family can cope.

Too Much Hair!

Q: Five years ago, at age 35, I had a hysterectomy. Shortly thereafter I noticed an increase in my facial hair, not only more and longer facial hair, but a stubblelike beard on my chin. I can tweeze the hair, but it is a daily task and I am never rid of it. Chemical hair removers cause a quite severe irritation on my face. Is there anything I can do to get *rid* of this hair safely?

A: Recent articles in various dermatologic and other medical publications have indicated that several drugs may be useful in the reduction of this coarse chin hair on women. One is spironolactone, used for this purpose in twenty patients. The study was published in the 1982 *Journal of the American Medical Association*; of the twenty patients treated, nineteen had a clearly beneficial reduction of the quantity of facial hair and a change to a more desirable soft, white facial hair.

Spironolactone is a potent diuretic (water pill) used in conditions such as fluid retention and high blood pressure. It causes potassium retention and therefore should not be used without follow-up by a dermatologist and/or an internal medicine specialist.

Other drugs for reducing facial hair include a fairly new one used mainly for the treatment of ulcer disease: cimetidine (Tagamet). It was noted that certain estrogenic effects took place with cimetidine, such as a slight increase in breast growth in men taking high doses. It then was theorized that it could reduce facial hair growth in women. This appears to have been the case. After eight or nine months, most female patients notice a decrease in the amount of facial hair, though not complete obliteration of it.

DERMALERT

Two medicines—spironolactone and cimetidine—appear to inhibit coarse hair growth on the faces of women. The medicines, however, must be taken for eight or nine months before an effect is seen, and the most noticeable effect is seen in patients with numerous dark hairs.

The problem with cimetidine is that it is *very expensive* and the drug needs to be continued for a long time before any effect is seen. Why? Remember those three cycles of head hair growth? Facial hairs cycle in an eight- to ten-month anagen-catagen-telogen phase. This means that any effect will not be seen until the hairs normally fall out, usually some time after that eight- to ten-month time period.

This is another case in which a drug (Tagamet) is not yet FDA-approved for correcting hair loss. In a small number of patients, side effects have included mild and transient diarrhea, dizziness, somnolence, rash, headache, and rare cases of fever.

DERMALERT

The growth cycle of facial hairs lasts some eight or nine months, so any medicine for decreasing hairs

would not be expected to show any change prior to
that time.

Recent talks by experts at dermatologic hair meetings indicate that
chronic epilation (pulling out hairs) may result in a permanent
decrease in the number of hairs. That is, if hairs are waxed or
tweezed time and again, numbers of them actually do not grow
back.

So you have several options open to you. You can continue
tweezing and waxing, which actually is a very effective way of
hair removal (albeit sometimes quite painful). You can bleach the
hairs so that they are less noticeable, which has worked well for
thousands of women. (This is best done with commercially available hair bleach. It's usually not irritating, if you carefully follow
the instructions on the type you purchase.)

Electrolysis is the *least* desirable way to remove hairs. I've seen
complications all too frequently from electrolysis, such as scarring
and infection. Besides these problems, electrolysis really doesn't
work as it's supposed to. Only a small fraction of the hairs are
actually destroyed, and aberrant hairs can result if only part of
the follicle is burned. These hairs grow crookedly into the surrounding skin, instead of out of the follicle opening, and severe
inflammation can result.

Q: I have lots of facial hair and cannot afford to have it removed professionally. What do you think of home electrolysis
machines? Are they safe?

A: Not only are they unsafe, but they're not very effective.
It's nearly impossible to guide one of these instruments down the
hair shaft the required distance to the hair bulb and burn out the
hair bulb accurately.

Q: Not too long ago, I heard you talking about a safe hair
removal system for the face. What is it?

A: That was the Nudit system of hair removal, but Nair,
Neet, and other barium sulfide-type agents can also work. Magic
Shave and Surgex are okay, but if your skin becomes irritated by
such agents they should be discontinued. It usually is wise to use
any depilatory only every third day or so, depending on tolerance.
Test any such product on a *small* patch of skin, before using it on
widespread areas.

Q: I'd like to know if depilatories are safe to use on your face over a number of years. Do lotions like this make the hair come in faster or thicker?

A: They are safe to use for years, and they do not change the character of the hair.

Q: Do hair removal creams remove the hair for good or does it come back? Does bleach remove the hair? Where can I buy these?

A: Hair removal creams remove the hair at the surface or just barely below it and are very satisfactory for those who are not irritated by them. It does not remove the hair for good, however. Bleach only changes the color of the hair and not its character or length. You can buy these concoctions in drugstores or the cosmetic sections of most department stores.

Q: My girlfriend has three or four moles on her face. They each have four long dark hairs growing out of them. Is there a safe product available to remove these hairs? Will it remove all the fuzz from her face?

A: The best thing to do with mole hairs is to pull them. You may have heard folklore that pulling hairs in moles causes skin cancer, but listen to the facts: hairs are not the substance of a mole and pulling the hair has no effect on the mole.

If your friend chooses a chemical hair remover, it will remove the fine fuzzy hair too.

Q: Does pulling facial hairs make them coarse and ugly?

A: No, pulling hairs does not cause them to become darker or coarser when they grow back in. The only animal in whom pulling out hairs changes it in any way is the rat: it stimulates growth.

One can even shave the face, and it won't change the character of the hair. I know that almost every woman reading this will think I'm crazy, but the facts are the facts. After all, how in the world could shaving off the top of a hair change the way the hair grows some two millimeters below the surface? If it did coarsen hair, bald men would *shave their heads* each morning to induce it to grow thicker.

Q: What can I do to remove a few dark hairs from the side of my upper lip?

A: Pluck them.

Q: Is there any risk of damaging the skin when the hair is pulled?

A: Essentially no. There are some cases of minor folliculitis (infections around hairs) after epilation, but this is rare. In some salons where waxing is done, an antibiotic ointment is used. This is probably worthwhile in preventing infection. If you're worried about this, try bacitracin ointment after plucking.

DERMALERT

Feel free to pull, clip, cut, shave, chemically remove, or wax facial hairs without fear of changing their character. The old wives' tale about the increasing coarseness of hair after a woman shaves is based only on the fact that the short stubble of hair which regrows out of the tiny follicle has a stiffer feel to it. After the hair gets long again, it's as soft as it was originally.

Q: Is there a selective hair removal process that is (1) permanent, (2) painless or nearly painless, and (3) safe?

A: No.

Q: I will soon be 30. Since my children were born, I have noticed facial hair growth which I am sure must be hormonal. What can be done about this?

A: Although the hair removal methods cited earlier may help you get rid of your coarse hair, some people get hair growth because they have a true endocrine gland (hormone-secreting) disease. Therefore, it is essential if you've noticed the onset of new hair growth to visit an endocrinologist or dermatologist for an evaluation of your gland system.

Q: You mentioned a high blood pressure medicine which might increase hair growth (minoxidil). I am taking hydrochlorothiazide. Is this the same one you were mentioning? I am also taking Aristocort in four-milligram tablets, and I have been having excess hair growth on my face. Is there a possibility that the Aristocort is doing it?

A: Hydrochlorothiazide should not have the hair growth effect, but Aristocort, being a cortisone-type medication, can certainly produce excess hair growth. You don't tell me what you're taking Aristocort for, but I would advise you to ask your physician about this. He or she might want to try having you off the Aristocort for a short time to see what happens to the hair on your face.

Be warned, however, that you may need the Aristocort for some medical disorder and the removal of it from your regimen should be the decision of your physician.

Q: I am a 30-year-old married male with tremendous amounts of hair all over my body. What makes hair grow so thickly on my back? What can I do to get rid of the hair for good (and *cheaply*)?

A: Your problem, a very rare complaint, is a tough one to handle, because the removal of such widespread areas of hair growth by waxing or plucking is not only tedious, but can result in superficial infection of the involved skin. As I've said previously, I do not recommend electrolysis. Shaving's possible, but the itching, when the hair begins to regrow, can be extreme. I guess, if asked to write the bottom line on your problem, since we all expect a man to be hairy in the areas which are currently bothering you, I'd encourage you to try to live with it. There just isn't an easy solution to your problem. If your friends call you "Gorilla," just tell them the heavy hair growth means you've got a lot of "virility hormone" around.

As you can see from the questions I've received on hair care, every person on earth is concerned about having or not having hair. It has become, and understandably so, a crucial part of our everyday lives. And yearly, we spend billions of dollars caring for our "strands of dead protein."

11

Nothing Stops Dandruff Like a Dark Blue Suit!

"Just look at this," said Candace as she moved her long brown hair off her dandruff-speckled sweater, "have you ever seen it this bad before? I keep hoping it'll snow every day, so people won't know about my problem."

When I looked at all the scales on her shoulders, I was reminded of my mentor, Dr. Glenn Marsh, who used to say, "Nothing stops dandruff like a dark blue suit!" In fact, Candace had not been able to wear blue for years, because of her dandruff.

Dandruff

What would you say if I told you everybody's *got* to have dandruff? Yep! That's right! Everybody. If we didn't, our scalps would be ten feet thick! You see, the skin remakes itself from top to bottom every twenty-eight days, so all that dead stuff's got to go somewhere. That's what the flakes are. The actual process is called *seborrhea*, or running of oil.

We think that scalp oil irritates the surface of the skin after it's secreted. As a parallel, consider stomach acid. If stomach acid remains in the stomach, no harm done. But if the acid regurgitates into the esophagus, or food tube, we feel the burning irritation as "heartburn." The situation is similar with dandruff and the worse form, seborrheic (seb-oh-REE-ick) dermatitis. The sebaceous oil is nonirritating while it's inside the oil gland, but does in fact irritate when it lies upon the scalp.

I'm constantly amazed, in my day-to-day practice of dermatology, how many people feel that washing the hair is somehow harmful. It's not. In fact, most people don't wash their hair enough to keep the oil removed efficiently. Amazingly, I've had numbers of patients who wash their hair only every *two* weeks or less, and a few who, because of especially difficult hair styles, wash only once monthly! Imagine the tremendous amount of oil which is held onto or near the scalp. This much scalp oil can be very irritating.

Q: My scalp is very dry and flaky, like dandruff, but it seems to be a lot worse. It is not like you see flakes on my shoulders— it seems to stick more to the scalp. My wife says that when my hair gets dirty, usually two days after I wash it, is has an awful odor. I am 30 years old and in good physical health. Can you treat my scalp?

A: You've obviously got the more severe type of seborrhea, called *seborrheic dermatitis*. This condition is accompanied by scalp irritation and redness with severe scaling. It takes special medications, including more potent tar shampoos and often topical cortisone, to get this under control. The odor is caused by bacteria which build up in the excess scalp oil characteristic of this condition. It's most effectively relieved by frequent washing, usually once daily.

Seborrheic dermatitis often starts in the late teens and early twenties. It's much more common in men than in women. Often it spreads from the scalp to the sides of the nose, eyebrows, and even the breastline area.

Your remark about the scales which "stick more to the scalp" is worrisome. That sounds as though it might be psoriasis. Be sure to read Chapter 16 to find out all about it.

Q: Is there anything that worsens dandruff, such as wearing a hat?

A: Not washing your hair will increase your dandruff, but wearing a hat will never affect it one way or the other. That's just another old skin myth.

Treatments for Seborrheic Dermatitis

Q: Please comment on "pH balance" of shampoos in relation to control of dandruff. Should hair products have a certain pH?

A: pH is an indicator of acidity. A low pH shampoo is more acid and theoretically is better for your hair. I would search for a fairly low pH shampoo, such as Dermalab X5T or Ionil T Plus, if I had seborrheic dermatitis, because not only does it have a nice low pH, but the tar and salicylic acid in it are extremely effective scale removers in seborrhea and seborrheic dermatitis. If you don't have a particular scalp condition, Phacid is the all-time best and mildest shampoo.

DERMALERT

Dermalab X5T and Ionil T Plus shampoo are two of the best treatments for mild seborrheic dermatitis.

Q: Could you tell me about the value of grenz rays on seborrheic dermatitis, compared to other treatments?

A: Grenz rays are a form of soft x-ray used in dermatology as an anti-inflammatory agent; that is, they decrease irritation in the upper layers of the skin. They penetrate very little. They're not harmful, like regular x-rays, when the dosage is administered properly, but these days, everyone is so afraid of the word "x-ray" that fewer and fewer dermatologists use the grenz technique anymore. Since we have effective forms of cortisone and tar preparations available, there's not much reason to.

Q: My problem concerns my ears. I have crusty ears and the doctor finally told me he thought it was a *skin* problem. They crust over and flake off and I've tried creams, drops, and shots, but the condition still comes back. A hearing specialist said my hearing was okay, but he could not do anything for my actual ear skin. Can you help me?

A: Flaky ears with a lot of itching is a regular characteristic of seborrheic dermatitis. But it can also happen in psoriasis and other diseases, so be sure to check with your dermatologist to make sure.

One of the main conditions we worry about in the ears, when they've been treated with multiple medicines, is allergic contact dermatitis. That is, you could possibly have gotten allergic to one or more of the ingredients of the medicines you've been using to treat your ear canals.

Be sure to read the discussion of the treatment of ear canals in Chapter 16, "Beating Psoriasis—How to Live without Leaving a Trail of Scales!" The technique which employs Halog solution on a Q-tip is the most effective I've ever found for handling ear canal rashes. As far as something you could get without a prescription, I doubt anything like Cortaid solution is anywhere near strong enough to help.

Q: Would it be permissible to use gentian violet on a Q-tip to get rid of a scaliness and flakiness in my ears? It doesn't hurt. I was told this might be good to use. What do you think?

A: If you don't mind having purple ears, gentian violet may actually help some itchy conditions, and it has mild antiyeast activity, but yeasts don't cause seborrheic dermatitis anyway. It probably just masked the scaliness so the patient didn't have to look at it while it healed *itself*. Forget it!

Q: I am convinced that seborrheic dermatitis is a contagious disease, and I'm afraid to tell the patrons in my hair design shop that they have it. They'll naturally know where they caught it— my shop! Please let me know, is this contagious?

A: Don't be afraid to tell your patrons they should see a dermatologist if you think they need to. Seborrheic dermatitis is no more contagious than freckles or a big nose. I'd sure hate to think that your customers are that narrow-minded. Maybe you've underestimated them. They deserve the service you can provide by helping them get a medical disorder checked out.

DERMALERT

Even severe dandruff is not contagious.

In fact, I have diagnosed several patients with severe skin cancers who came to me for help because of thoughtfulness of hairdressers, beauticians, and barbers alert to their customers' real needs. You're a professional, so get out there and give professional advice! Certainly you can't make diagnoses or give treatment, but you can recommend dermatologic care when and if something looks unusual.

DERMALERT

If your barber or a stylist notices a lesion or spot of concern in your scalp, have your dermatologist check it immediately. It may save your skin.

Now that you realize that all scalps have dandruff, you'll be better equipped to seek help if the condition progresses. With the shampoos and medicines available today, no one needs to put up with "snowy shoulders." If your scaling and itching problem is severe, relief is as close as your dermatologist's office.

12

Her Skin

"I'm sorry, Doctor," said a patient, Jenny, "but a woman's skin is just not like a man's skin! My face is too dry to use regular acne lotions. I *need* a moisturizer. I *need* cosmetics. And for you to tell me that I cannot use them just will not work for me!" That statement, from an irate patient, expresses much of the bewilderment of women who encounter the advice and regulations of traditional dermatology. When, as a resident, I overheard her saying this in the office of a private dermatologist, I realized that not enough dermatologists think to give female skin the very special care it needs.

In this chapter, I will touch on many topics which have been traditionally only skimmed over by dermatologists, since we are mainly concerned with treating diseases rather than with the cosmetic needs of patients. But persons like Jenny, I found out, need special handling, diseased or not.

We know a lot about the peculiar mix of hormones and genes which surround and affect the skin of a woman. Many of the problems mentioned in this chapter affect women exclusively, but others also affect men. They are mentioned here because, in my experience, they are far more common in women. Take pigmentation, for example, an area where hormonal influences exert maximal effect.

Melasma and Other Pigment Problems

Thousands of women develop "pigmentation brown spots"—melasma—on their faces during their teens, twenties, and thirties. These annoying flat, tannish blotches can literally disfigure a woman, making normal social life virtually impossible. This so-called mask of pregnancy can make a woman look like a raccoon. Dermatologists think this altered pigmentation results from the hormone changes that accompany childbearing. Unfortunately, the mask of pregnancy is also a severe occasional side effect of taking birth control pills.

The actual brownish facial color of melasma results from deposition of excess color pigment, melanin, in the upper layer of skin, the epidermis. Unfortunately, most cases of melasma fade extremely slowly, if at all. Some women notice very slight fading with time, but I've seen the problem persist for *years* without any visible lightening.

Let's look at melasma and some other common pigment problems with "her skin."

Q: I am 38 years old, and I have quite a bit of pigment on my face. Are there any creams or new treatments to clear it up?

A: For years women have turned toward over-the-counter creams to fade their facial pigment. These creams contain a minuscule amount of hydroquinone, a chemical which slows the output of melanin from the tiny skin pigment cells. However, the concentration of hydroquinone is so slight in these "medicines" that they take months to years to work, if indeed they ever do. In practice, they often don't. At least I've never seen a case of melasma clear up with these over-the-counter fade creams.

DERMALERT

Over-the-counter fade creams are useless for removing pigment abnormalities.

Dermatologists have found that certain agents such as ammo-
niated mercury (used much less than previously, because it can
irritate) and vitamin A acid (Retin-A) mixed with cortisone cream,
can lighten these areas.

Recently, a more effective remedy has been developed by the
Neutrogena Corporation (the same company that makes Neutrogena soap for irritated or sensitive skin). The new agent is called
Melanex. It's concentrated hydroquinone in a specially formulated
lotion which penetrates to the exact level of the skin where the
pigment is made. Supplied in a convenient pad-topped bottle, it's
designed to be applied sparingly to the skin twice daily. To this
date, it's the most effective depigmenting lotion I've ever seen.
It's a prescription item, however, so you'll have to ask your dermatologist for it and for careful instructions on its use.

DERMALERT

Melanex, a new compound by Neutrogena, can safely
lighten most cases of the mask of pregnancy.

An important study in the *British Journal of Dermatology* in 1981
showed that doctors can often predict how well a patient would
improve on hydroquinone therapy by testing her with a black
light called a Wood's light. In most cases this light reveals whether
you have the epidermal (surface) type of pigment or the dermal
(deep) type. The former responds much better to Melanex than
the latter. Ask your doctor if he or she uses this test. It'll give
you some indication of how well you can expect to improve.

Q: I have the mask of pregnancy, but I've never taken birth
control pills, nor have I ever been pregnant. Why do I have this
problem?

A: That's a tough one. It seems that, in some people, the
pigment cells are exquisitely sensitive to the effect of sex hor-

mones. That means that even women who have not been pregnant may have enough of the required hormone around, possibly
progesterone, to turn on their melanocytes.

Believe it or not, there are even some *men* who have melasma!
And certainly they don't take the pill. But, as you know from our
discussion of hormones in Chapter 7, each of us has both male
and female hormones. In those men with melasma, their tiny
amounts of estrogen or progesterone must be just enough to turn
on their facial color cells.

Q: My brown facial patches are much worse in the summer.
They fade almost completely in the winter months. Why do I
worsen in summer?

A: Ah, yes, the sun! You know already, of course, how dermatologists feel about sun exposure on faces. But in the treatment
of melasma, avoidance of sun exposure is not only important but
crucial! I have *never* seen a patient's melasma improve without
her taking great pains to keep the sun's rays off her face.

How do you avoid it? Sunscreens are essential. Melasma patients should use these lotions every day, because even the small
amount of sunlight gotten going to and from the house and car
can maintain the ugly pigment. In Chapter 17, you'll learn a lot
more about protection from the sun in ways which really will save
your skin.

Breast Skin Cysts

Q: I've got what my doctor calls epidermoid cysts just beneath the skin, around my breasts. Could they be related to nursing? Diet?

A: Occasionally a woman will develop a few plugged oil glands
around the areolae, or brown areas of the nipples, usually in
response to nursing an infant. These are quite normal, if they're
not excessively large, and sometimes will go away without treatment. If they get large, sore, inflamed, or infected, they should
be examined by your physician. Antibiotics, surgery, or a combination may be needed to resolve them. Diet has nothing to do
with the development of these tiny cysts.

Pregnancy and Stretch Marks

Q: How long does it take for the skin to get back in shape after a pregnancy?

A: The tremendous elasticity of the skin has been a constant wonder for thousands of years. Imagine the incredible stretching force of the pregnant abdomen; it's a miracle that the baby doesn't stretch right through! The skin performs admirably in shrinking down after delivery, usually taking only a few days to get back most of its normal tone, but almost all women are left with some permanent stretching which will not go away.

Q: What is a "stretch mark"?

A: Stretch marks, or striae, are actual scars in the dermis, or second layer of the skin, in response to the stretching forces of pregnancy. When the collagen, the strong supporting network of the dermis, is pulled almost to the breaking point, the skin very wisely starts to lay down new layers of collagen fibers to add strength. This results in the classic stretch mark we all know and hate!

Of course, everyone knows about the stretch marks related to pregnancy, but many patients ask about the stretch marks most people get during the normal pubertal weight gain. These are usually around the hips and thighs, but can sometimes encircle the entire leg.

Another type of stretch mark is the type acquired by weight-lifters. These "starburst" striae radiate outward from the armpits, and progressively worsen as the weightlifter builds muscle mass in the shoulder areas.

One last type of stria deserves mentioning. If you develop reddish-purple stretch marks which don't ever fade back to the usual ivory white coloration, you should show them to your doctor. They could be a sign of a serious hormonal imbalance called Cushing's syndrome. Be sure you show this type of stretch mark to a physician.

Q: I'm pregnant right now and I've been getting an itchy rash on my stretch marks. Why?

A: Stretch marks commonly undergo some inflammation during their lifetimes. Usually, this is only a mild redness, but sometimes it's bad enough to cause quite a bit of itching. This is about equivalent to our grandparents saying that "if it's itching, it's healing," in that your body's trying to "heal" a dangerously stretched place in the skin. During this process, the contraction of the scarred stretch marks stimulates the itch fibers in the skin.

More important, the itching in stretch marks is often the result of an allergy to something being applied to the skin surface. This could be anything from an allergy to lanolin to a reaction to vitamin E, a frequent skin sensitizer.

Recently, there's been reported a curious "dermatosis of pregnancy," a rash acquired during pregnancy which involves striae exactly like yours. It's got the strange name of PUPPP, and we'll discuss it at more length shortly.

There's no magic cream or lotion you can apply to the skin which will correct stretch marks. If there were such ingredients, there'd be no striae!

Q: How *do* you get rid of stretch marks, then?

A: You don't. But they often become less obtrusive with time, and plastic surgeons can do wonders in hiding them. If yours really are noticeable, then you should consult a plastic surgeon. And remember Covermark! This remarkable makeup system, described in Chapter 3, is quite capable of hiding these unsightly marks, sometimes for days at a time.

Q: A friend of mine developed a case of what her doctor called PUPPP during her pregnancy. What's that?

A: The initials PUPPP stand for *p*ruritic *u*rticarial *p*apules and *p*laques of *p*regnancy. This is an extremely itchy rash which starts like a very severe case of hives over the thighs and abdomen during late pregnancy. In fact, it can *start* in and around stretch marks. It often looks like hives, with large accompanying flat spots. PUPPP itches like crazy! And it's this itching which usually bothers mothers-to-be enough that they seek treatment.

This particular rash doesn't affect the baby's health (nor does it apparently cause the *baby* to itch), but it is an awful nuisance.

The treatment for PUPPP is topical cortisone, usually in cream or lotion form. Extreme cases can be settled down with antihistamines, and even internal cortisone if the obstetrician and pediatrician agree it's okay. The rash goes away spontaneously at delivery or shortly thereafter, but you can get it again with your next child. We don't yet know the exact cause of PUPPP. Some factor produced by the baby or the placenta has been theorized as a cause, but never proved.

DERMALERT

Since the skin is such an excellent reflector of the body's internal systems, a pregnant woman should have any persistent itching or rash checked by her doctor.

Spider Veins

Q: When I was pregnant with my first child, I developed three red spots on my face. I read in an expectant mothers' magazine that these are broken capillaries, called *spiders*, and that they would go away after the baby was born. Well, I've had my *second* child and they are *still* there! Is there anything I can do to get rid of them? Would a cream skin lightener work?

A: You've just learned the cardinal rule of dermatology: If your disease hasn't read the textbook, it may not know how to act. In short, some go away, and some don't. Naturally, that is. Therapeutically, there's a whale of a lot of things you can do for vascular spiders besides cover them up (don't forget Covermark).

In most people (70 percent) spiders are the result of the small amount of natural estrogens in our systems. Circulating estrogen (a female hormone) can, under the right circumstances, activate tiny blood vessels to overgrow, forming a spider.

Women have more spiders than men because of their naturally higher estrogen levels, and these levels soar with pregnancy, causing even more of these little nuisances to form. The lucky women are those whose spots apparently *have* read the textbook, and actually go away after parturition.

Cream skin lighteners are worthless in removing these dilated, or expanded, capillaries. In fact, by slowly lightening the normal masking pigment overlying these lesions, one could imagine that they might even get worse.

Q: What causes the spider veins to *break*, then?

A: They're *not* broken! Blood is actively flowing through them constantly. Our next questioner demonstrates that. Read on, please.

DERMALERT

There's no such thing as a "broken blood vessel" on the face. Spider veins are intact, flowing blood vessels!

Q: I have red spots on my chest the size of quarters, and when pressed, they go away for an instant, and then turn immediately red again. Can they be removed?

A: Yes. Now that you know that these are *not* "broken" veins, you'll understand a lot better how we dermatologists treat them. Our first line of defense is the *electrodesiccator*, or electric needle. This fantastically useful machine can gently zap a spider vein with a small charge of electricity, sealing its fate permanently. The procedure stings a little, but it's worth it when you walk out of the office usually with no sign of those nasty little spiders (except possibly a little swelling where the vessel was zapped shut).

However, the human circulation is a marvelous machine. It seems to know where it wants blood to flow and will try hard to redrill a hole in the vessel. Usually this will occur within a few days, but may take as long as a month for the spider to start flowing again. If this happens, you'll have to have another treatment to seal it again.

Q: Is there anything more effective than electric needles to use on vascular spiders?

A: Not really. But there are some new techniques now being tested which indeed show definite promise.

Q: Do laser beams get rid of reddish-purple capillaries, and is there any permanent scarring? Is the method safe?

A: For the most part, lasers are not being used much for the destruction of single or several enlarged capillaries on the face. The most notable exception to this is the larger grossly expanded veins on the nose, which often accompany the middle age acnelike disease called *rosacea*. The most valuable use for the laser on the face is for people, usually rosacea victims, with totally red noses.

In these cases, the nose can be treated widely with the laser to seal almost all the superficial vessels simultaneously.

For tiny vessels, however, the risk of scarring, and leaving a mark which is worse than the original spider, is significant.

Don't Be Caught with a Red Face

Q: How else can I tone down the redness on my nose?

A: Try Borghese's Green Color Corrector Foundation. That's right, I said *green*! The reason behind this is simple: When the red on your nose and the makeup's green color combine, a flesh tone is produced. The color corrector is available at most cosmetic counters, and there are several other manufacturers who produce a green-tinted foundation.

Q: What causes capillary formation on the cheeks—anything besides female hormones?

A: You bet! Most of us in dermatology feel the sun is influential in the formation of them. We also know that the use of certain topical compounds for treatment of some skin problems of the face can make them appear. These topicals, called *fluorinated steroids*, are forms of cortisone with an attached fluoride molecule. The fluoride makes the creams about ten times more potent, but the subsequent higher potency can both induce thinning in the skin and cause tiny blood vessels to grow quite large. Therefore, I'm constantly on the lookout for patients using treatment creams which are fluorinated. Except in the most dire circumstances, they're rarely needed on soft facial, neck, or groin skin.

A large group of internal diseases, the so-called autoimmune diseases, such as lupus erythematosus, scleroderma, and so forth, can cause spiders. The take-home message here is that if you or any member of your family have *many* vascular spiders, you should be seen by an internist or rheumatologist, a specialist in sorting out these strange disorders.

DERMALERT

A large group of internal diseases can cause spider veins. If you have many spider veins, ask your doctor to examine you.

Q: Is a person with diabetes more likely to have broken capillaries than a nondiabetic patient?

A: Although there are those who think that diabetes is a disease closely coupled with blood vessel problems, diabetics are no more likely to have enlarged vascular spiders than the nondiabetic population.

Q: Can a very fair-skinned person with capillaries visible on the face have a face-lift? Would this be a cure for the red spidery look on the nose and face?

A: The number of capillaries on the face shouldn't affect one's possibilities for a face-lift at all. But I certainly wouldn't expect a face-lift to cure the spidery look, either.

Leg Spiders—a Tougher Problem

Q: My legs above the knees are full of broken spider veins, caused by "hard work." I used to love to go swimming, but now I'm ashamed to put on a suit, and for the last twenty years I've been ashamed even to put shorts on! Is there any help for my problem?

A: Veins on the legs are more a problem to dermatologists than veins in other locations. Maybe it's because of the vast numbers of them on the legs. Obliterating them all seems like an insurmountable task. I think they are technically harder to get rid of on the legs, too.

The problem seems to come from the actual anatomy of the leg veins. They are longer and of larger caliber than those we usually see on the face; so a single zap with the electric needle is a lot less likely to knock out a leg vein. When many tiny shocks are used, small dots may appear sometime thereafter, like tiny tracks left by the procedure. The process occasionally works excellently, but it's less a sure bet than the same technique used on the face.

DERMALERT

> Lasers and electrodesiccation (electric needle treatments) don't work as well for big leg veins as they do for facial spider veins.

Q: Is there a cover cream or cover-up treatment for these? I'm forty years old, and age is *not* helping me accept them any easier.

A: I'll risk repeating myself by referring you again to Chapter 3 where you can read in detail about the fabulous cover-up system called Covermark. It makes a spectacular leg makeup system, because it's *waterproof*! See, you can even be a bathing beauty again!

Q: Can lasers be used on the legs? How about the new "injections" for these veins that I've read about?

A: Again, although lasers indeed can obliterate these vessels, the treatment is far from perfect because of the scarring it leaves. We all had hope, when lasers were introduced, that they would solve some of these horrendous cosmetic problems, but, alas, such is not the case. The exception, of course, is the removal of tattoos (Chapter 13) and port-wine stains (Chapter 3), both of which are best treated by lasers.

I'm glad you asked about the injection therapy. This is one very promising avenue of treatment for medium-sized leg veins which does work, when performed by a dermatologist or surgeon skilled in the technique. The therapy consists of injecting a tiny quantity of strong salt solution into the vein. Incidentally, the needles used are so small that they are hardly visible, and a magnifying lens usually must be used with them.

The salt solution irritates the lining cells of the tiny blood vessels so much that the vessel dies and is digested (cleaned up) by the body's natural defenses, the white blood cells. While the technique *does* work, it takes a tremendously patient patient and a patient doctor (and sometimes even a patient doctor patient!). Also, the expense can be considerable, so investigate costs carefully before having your spots treated. Some dermatologists are so proficient at performing these little injections that they set aside whole *days* to do the procedure for the hordes of women desiring it. If your dermatologist or surgeon doesn't do these saline injections, as they are called, then you might ask him or her for a referral to one who does.

DERMALERT

Saline injection therapy can greatly reduce or eliminate enlarged capillaries and tiny "starburst" veins on the legs.

Don't Pore Over Your Pores

Q: What can be done for "enlarged pores" on the face? Is a scrub (gritty) cleanser, used daily, good for them?

A: Most enlarged pores on the facial skin are the result of one's unlucky ancestry more than anything else. And when you stop to think of how many thousands of women (and men) complain about their *own* enlarged pores, it's truly a wonder why we don't often see large pores on *others*! What I'm trying to explain is that pores are rarely, if ever, visible to other people, but in this day and age of the great "magnifying mirror" society, most people can enlarge their images enough to spot the proverbial "nit on a gnat"!

If you insist on having something done to enlarged pores, first try Clinique's fabulous Pore Minimizer Makeup. It's great for hiding pores and making you look a lot smoother than you think you are.

Cellulite—Great International Hoax

Q: I don't know if it is correct to ask a dermatologist about cellulite, but is there any way to get rid of this bumpy skin on my thighs, buttocks, and hips?

A: Cellulite is the greatest hoax ever perpetrated on the beauty-conscious American public. The very term "cellulite" even sounds like one's cells are contaminated with some modern pollutant. Cellulite is just a descriptive term for the way fat piles up in the supporting network of the skin. The more *fat*, the more *dimples*! The *less* fat, the *less* dimples. It's really as simple as that, but every time I tell audiences about the truth of the horrible and dreaded cellulite, I receive calls and letters by the hundreds, telling me what an iconoclast and beauty nihilist I am. Sorry, but truth's truth.

Q: Okay, then, what would one do to *stop* getting it?

A: Stop eating.

DERMALERT

Lose weight, lose cellulite! Simple!

Fat Suction—Not Necessarily the "Easy" Way

Q: On a television talk show you said that the best cure for cellulite was weight loss. I am fairly thin, but about two months ago I gained about ten pounds and the cellulite started to show up on my upper thighs. Please give me some advice as to what I can do to get rid of this ugly stuff, besides losing weight? Isn't there a new "suction" operation for this?

A: In this operation, fat cells are sucked out through a tube inserted in the skin through a small inconspicuous incision. While the technique sounds as if it has some merit, I'd hasten to add that some very severe complications can result. These include infection below the skin, hemorrhage, and disruption of the nerves, arteries, and veins which supply the involved skin. This could conceivably result even in the *death* of small or large patches of skin.

Ask your plastic surgeon specifically about his or her special competence in the suction operation: total number of cases, results, complications, and, most important, a list of patients your surgeon has operated on so you can *talk* to them personally and actually *see* the results.

DERMALERT

Beware of the new "fat suction" operation. You must find an expert with a *proven* track record first!

Freckles—Bane of the Bonnie Lass

Q: When I was 19, I got a pretty bad sunburn, which peeled and became raw and sore for a couple of weeks. When it healed, I had sun freckles on my chest, shoulders, back, and even on my abdomen. They're not very dark, but they bother me. I'm 25 now, and even though I am fairly attractive, I feel very self-conscious about wearing sundresses and some other summer fashions. Can you help me?

A: Sun freckling is a problem many women (and men) face in their search for a tan. Even short, intense exposures to the sun can change the skin's texture and color forever. In your case, it turned on a host of freckles from the superficial pigment layer of the epidermis.

Treatment? That all depends on how many freckles you have and upon the amount of pain you're willing to go through to have them removed. My patient Wanda sounded just like you.

"Help me get these nasty freckles off, Dr. Bark!" she exclaimed.

"I'd love to," I said, "but you know that involves freezing them all with liquid nitrogen?"

"Sure, go to it," she said. She slid out of her shirt, revealing a whole forest of brown freckles of every size and shape. She looked like a leopard!

"Uh, where would you like me to start freezing?"

"Gosh, I don't know," she said. "Maybe if you'd just get a fifty-five-gallon drum of the stuff, you could hold me by the heels and just *dip* me in!"

It would have been a mammoth job indeed. We decided to frost the biggest and most objectionable ones lightly, leaving her "adolescents" to grow up a little before we chill them off. I'm sure she'll be back, on and off for years, because of her sun indiscretions.

DERMALERT

Isolated freckles can usually be removed nicely by cryosurgery (liquid nitrogen freezing treatments).

Corns and Footwear—Ah, There's the Rub

Q: What can you do about my soft corns between my little toes and the next ones? Could my shoes have something to do with them forming? I have several pairs which seem to irritate them.

A: A wonderful podiatrist who used to treat my mother's soft corns used to say, "The poor feet! Whenever you realize you *have* feet, there's almost always something wrong with them!" And he was right. Tight footwear is the main reason for the formation of soft corns. It seems that, in the search for fashion, we've created several new diseases, not the least of which are these nasty little nuisances called "soft corns."

Whenever two toes are pushed together, as they are most effectively with tight footwear, the skin begins to thicken to protect and cushion the bones below. But the poor skin, just doing its faithful job of protecting our innards, doesn't realize that the thickening will eventually hurt and greatly irritate the skin itself. Correction of the problem depends on relieving the pressure of the narrow footwear while treating the corns.

DERMALERT

The real secret to banishing soft corns forever is the elimination of tight footwear.

Treating them is much easier said than done, however. Some people can get relief by just putting cotton pads, or even "dough-nut"-type adhesive bandages around the corns to better distribute the pressure over a larger area. Often, however, it's necessary to use a mild salicylic acid plaster (available at foot care counters) to soften and gently coax the thick part of the corn off the tender skin below. Follow the directions on the package very carefully, especially the advice concerning diabetic foot care, because *no* diabetic should undergo any foot treatment without his or her doctor's advice.

DERMALERT

Diabetics should never treat their own feet without the specific advice of their endocrinologist, diabetol-ogist, internist, or family physician. Diabetic skin heals more slowly than normal skin.

The Eyes Have It!

Q: Would you please discuss mascara and eye shadow in relation to the health of the skin?

A: Several years ago researchers discovered that mascara (as well as other cosmetics) could become rancid with time. Bacteria were overgrowing in the cosmetics! Since this could possibly infect the eyes, users were warned to replace their mascara on a regular basis.

DERMALERT

Get new eye cosmetics every three months to prevent eye infections.

However, eye infections did indeed begin to show up, and these were occasionally traced to a very bad practice at cosmetic counters. We've all seen demonstration cosmetics displayed in women's areas of department stores. These are being used by many different women, thus causing many possible strains of bacteria to collect in the demonstration unit. Ophthalmologists (physicians specializing in eye care) warned the public about the possible contamination, and encouraged cosmetic companies to distribute individual, single-use packets of "tester" cosmetics. If the practice somehow reaches mascara, or if salespeople will just not permit the testing of mascara, the infection problem may be greatly lessened.

DERMALERT

Never use anyone else's eye cosmetics. To do so is to risk the very eyes with which you're reading this.

Eye infection is not the sole worry in regard to mascara. Leading dermatologists and eye care doctors specializing in cosmetic problems have warned that the mascara brushes themselves can cause damage and embed dangerous bacteria into the cornea (clear part of the eye), if the eye is touched. So the recommendation is that one should *never* touch the eyeball itself with any cosmetic applicator.

Women should *never* apply eye cosmetics in moving vehicles. One famous dermatologist recently remarked that she actually saw a woman at a stoplight drive away when the light changed, while simultaneously applying her mascara. (As yet no word has been received on whether she incurred any traffic injuries!)

DERMALERT

Never apply eye cosmetics in a moving vehicle. Serious corneal scratches could result.

Q: Some women apply eye cosmetics to the very edge of their lids. Is this safe?

A: Absolutely not! Applying eyeliner to the extreme edge of the lid *inside* the lash line, is the most dangerous of all eye cosmetic application techniques. At the moment the liner is being applied to the lid line, the brush is its absolute closest to the eyeball. Also, the liner itself, if contaminated, has an excellent chance of getting into the eye directly. The look is alluring, but it may lure you into some very sight-threatening eye diseases.

DERMALERT

Save your precious eyes. Never apply eyeliner to the extreme edge of the lid *inside* the lash line.

Q: What causes the dark circles under and around my eyes? Is there any way to get rid of them?

A: For years I didn't think dark circles under eyes really existed, or if they did exist, that they certainly wouldn't fluctuate with tiredness, etc., the way people said they did. But I recently heard an excellent professional talk by an allergist who had studied this condition extensively, and he had an interesting explanation for the darkness.

The eyes, and the bony orbits which hold them, have extensive blood circulation in and around them. On the upper cheeks and lower lids, these vessels form a plexus, or weblike network, just under the translucent skin. The skin is so thin in this area that they can actually be seen. As a person grows tired during a long day, or if he or she has sinusitis or allergies, the blood circulating through these vessels slows down and dilates the veins wide open. The bluish color shines through, then, making what appears to be a "dark circle" under the eye.

DERMALERT

Dark circles under the eyes are a part of your anatomical makeup. While they can't be eliminated, cosmetics can make them invisible.

There's no really good way to get rid of them, but they are not as likely to be prominent if you've had enough rest, and if you don't have sinusitis or allergies. Cosmetics work wonders here, and again, Covermark leads the pack with its terrific ability to hide unsightly spots on the skin.

Astringents

Q: Several cosmetic companies sell "oil control" liquids to be put on after astringents and before makeup. Are these products supposed to inhibit the appearance of shine on the skin for a long time? Are they harmful?

A: That's what they're *supposed* to do, all right, but in practice, there's really nothing that can stop oil from being secreted by the skin (that is, with the exception of Accutane, the new acne medicine which actually does stop it). So you're really left with removing the oil as it forms with astringents, like the ones you mentioned, or by covering up the oil with absorbent powders.

The products you mention are not harmful; they just don't really do what they claim to do. They remove surface oil only.

Cosmetics and Skin Cancer

Q: Is there any connection between skin cosmetics and cancer?

A: Yes. The first prevents the second. For instance, because they wear lipstick, women have an almost negligible incidence of lip cancer. It stops the harmful, cancer-causing rays of the sun from striking the lips. The same can be true for the rest of the face, especially if one of the newer, sunscreen-containing cosmetics, such as Dermage, is used. (Dermage is available only at your dermatologist's office.)

Aloe—Just Another Gimmick

Q: Are aloe vera products good for the skin?

A: There's really no good evidence one way or the other, that the aloe vera (the "burn plant") juice actually does any harm *or* good. It's been rumored for years that it was good to break open the thick leaves of this plant and apply the juice to minor burns or other injuries. But studies that would show the efficacy or nonefficacy of this substance have not yet been done.

"Skin Writing"

Q: I have an unusual problem. I buy good jewelry, but I constantly have black discoloration of my skin under the metal frames of my glasses where they touch my cheeks, and under my rings, which are made of silver and gold. What chemical in my skin causes this to happen just to me?

A: To me, this is one of the most fascinating stories in all of dermatology. First, it doesn't happen just to you, but to thousands of women. Second, no skin chemical is responsible for this discoloration. Third, your silver and gold rings probably are the fine metals you think they are. The *real* problem is your *face powder!*

Let me explain. Jewelry metals are usually fairly soft. But face powders contain extremely hard, tiny, sharp flakes of metals such as titanium, which are much harder than the metals in your jewelry. The friction of your glass rims upon the powder on your cheeks, and of the rings on the fingers of the hands which applied the powder, actually causes infinitesimal particles of gold or silver to be abraded from both glasses and rings. Why doesn't the abraded metal look gold or silver in color, then? Because the particles are so tiny that they won't accurately reflect light much at all. They just scatter it. Therefore, taken together, they look black. And for that reason, the problem has been named *black dermographism*, which means "black-colored skin writing."

So how does a woman get around this unsightly problem? Simple! Try not to get *any* powder on the cheek areas which contact the rims of your glasses. And don't fail to *wash your hands* thoroughly after each use of your face powder. The problem will leave you instantly.

DERMALERT

If you have problems with blackish discolorations under your fine jewelry, keep your face powder and other cosmetics away from the area, and the problem will stop.

Cosmetic Allergies

Q: I have had an itchy rash on my face most of the time for about six months. But I've been using the same cosmetics for *years!*

A: That statement, "But I've used it for years, so I couldn't be allergic to it," is the most common remark of patients with cosmetic allergy. It's also the most inaccurate. The skin, magnificent organ that it is, can learn how to become allergic to a substance even after years of using it without problems. In dermatology, we see this happen constantly.

DERMALERT

Don't think that if you've used a product for a long time, you can't be allergic to it. The skin can become allergic to a substance *any time!*

A patient named Meri sought my help with a chronically swollen eyelid. She had used the same cosmetics for many years, and had had this facial reaction for only a month. As a busy young executive, she had not had the time to get the problem checked out earlier.

When we patch-tested her to the standard American Academy of Dermatology (AAD) kit of allergens, she showed a strong positive reaction to formalin, a substance usually used as a preservative. Looking through Meri's cosmetics revealed that her *nail polish* contained (at that time) formalin.

"I'll bet you're in one heck of a hurry most of the time, right?" I asked.

"Sure, Dr. Bark. I always seem to have ten things on my schedule, and nine of them are overdue."

"Put your nail polish on in a hurry, too?"

"Usually. It's a quick job in the mornings."

"Aha!" I exclaimed. "That's where you're getting the formalin."

"Beg your pardon?"

"You see, Meri," I explained, "when you run out of the house with slighty soft nail polish, you've been touching your lids occasionally. This leaves traces of the very material you're allergic to right on your poor eyelids. And that's what's causing your dermatitis."

"Fantastic!" she said. "But does that mean that I can never again wear my favorite nail polish?"

"No, not at all. All you have to do to make sure you don't react to it is to be absolutely sure that the polish is *dry* when you are ready to go in the morning. And to make sure of that, all you have to do is the 'dry test.' "

"I give up," she said, "what's the dry test?"

"Just touch a cotton ball lightly to the nails when you think they're dry. If *any* fibers from the cotton are left on the nail, then you'll have to give it more time. Be sure to do this when you have some extra time, so that you can get an idea how long it takes to really get your polish dry."

Meri's problem disappeared, and she was able to continue using the polish. She also took care to avoid other substances with formalin, such as some shampoos, certain toothpastes, permanent-press fabrics, and so forth.

Q: I developed an allergy on my face to a cortisone cream I was using for dry skin. When will the allergy be out of my system?

A: Actually, if you've really got an allergy to some component of that cream, you'll probably never lose it. That type of allergy is mediated, or caused, by certain cells in your body called *lymphocytes*. This type of white blood cell is especially competent at picking up substances or chemicals from outside the body and recognizing them as "foreign." And, good little police officers that they are, the lymphocytes react against anything recognized in such a way by forming antibodies. They, in turn, cause the red, itchy rash to occur.

Antibodies are the tremendous protective chemicals which keep all of us alive each day by fighting off all sorts of infections, eliminating some microscopic malignancies, and performing a million other functions we never think about.

DERMALERT

Once allergic, always allergic!

Q: I get a horrible reaction to my brand of lipstick—my lips suppurated for a long time and I couldn't wear *any* lipstick for a couple of years without my lips splitting, cracking, and bleeding. What could have caused this?

A: Sounds like a classic case of allergy to one or more ingredients in the lipstick. Your body recognized some part of the lipstick formula as a foreign substance and reacted against it. Some women accurately recognize the allergy has occurred and switch lipsticks, hoping to avoid it. What is not often realized is that many lipsticks, and other cosmetics for that matter, have common ingredients, especially the preservatives, which frequently cause allergy.

The real key is to be patch-tested to find out the exact chemical which has caused the allergy. Then you can carefully pick your next lipstick to exclude that chemical.

Important: the ingredients of cosmetics are sometimes *changed* without notice from the manufacturer. This is another reason you could get allergic to a cosmetic you've used for some time.

Nickel Allergies—A Problem That Shows Your True Mettle

Q: I've got a problem wearing most types of jewelry. I get all itchy around my earlobes every time I put in my pierced earrings, and my neck goes crazy with a rash every time I try to wear my good necklaces. Should I just give up?

A: Absolutely not! It sounds like you have "nickel allergy." This is almost always the problem when a jewelry rash is acquired. You tipped me off to the diagnosis yourself when you mentioned that you wear *pierced* earrings. That's where most women first come into contact with the element nickel, and that's where the lymphocytes first pick it up and recognize it as a foreign substance.

DERMALERT

What sometimes starts off looking like a minor infection on the earlobe after piercing is usually the first sign of nickel dermatitis, a horrible, lifelong problem.

Once again, the real shame is that if you get allergic to nickel, you're apt to be allergic to it for a long, long time. A lab technician named Julie at the Medical College of Georgia developed nickel allergy after getting her ears pierced in a shopping center. Since she had to deal with metals such as nickel in the lab all day, Julie was really in trouble.

Unluckily, she demonstrated a fact about nickel allergy that no one likes to think about. Unlike other allergies which fade rather rapidly once the offending allergen or chemical is removed, Julie's rash hung on for *months* after a single exposure. Nickel binds to the upper skin layers, thus causing extended dermatitis.

What could we do for Julie? We tried everything to get her back into wearing her favorite earrings. Some of our methods worked, and others did not.

Whenever possible, we asked Julie not to wear her earrings. This helped somewhat by limiting her exposure to the offending metal. We coated them with clear nail polish, so that the nickel would not contact her skin so easily, when she absolutely had to wear them.

We treated her with a medicine called Kenalog spray, which leaves a resin behind to coat the ear hole and protect it from the nickel. Kenalog spray also contains a potent cortisone which treats the rash.

We tested all her jewelry items with a chemical test kit available to all dermatologists, called the *dimethylglyoxime* (DMG) kit, which revealed that several other items were nickel-positive. We eliminated these from her contact as well.

DERMALERT

The DMG kit, available at your dermatologist's office, may be used to test your jewelry for the presence of nickel.

Since all our efforts were only partially successful, we asked a local jeweler to replace Julie's DMG-positive earring posts with ones made of surgical grade stainless steel, the only metal universally safe to wear by those allergic to nickel. It contains nickel, but it's so tightly bound into the alloy that it can't escape to cause dermatitis. That's when we residents discovered a much easier way to get Julie back into earrings and jewelry again. At the American Academy of Dermatology meeting one December, I found a display by a little company in New York which makes very nice, certified nickel-free, hypoallergenic earrings and other jewelry, called Ear-Eze. Their address is:

Ear-Eze H & A Enterprises, Inc.
143-19 25th Avenue P.O. Box 489
Whitestone, New York 11357

These folks are very cooperative in supplying nickel-free items directly to patients. Write them, and they'll send you an order form for their beautiful set of color catalogs.

Since an ounce of prevention is worth a pound of cure, women should take care to ensure that the *original* piercing of their ears is done with completely nickel-free materials. My dermatology professor used to dread nickel dermatitis so much that when young ladies would ask him if he'd pierce their ears, he'd say, "Sure, I'll pierce your ears, if you'll let me put a ring in your nose at the same time!"

While we have come a long way since then, I still insist that completely nickel-free posts be used. And you don't find those very often at department store piercing salons. You may, however, convince them to let you take the piercing posts to your dermatologist so they can be tested for the presence of nickel. It's simple, and should definitely be done first, to make sure your posts are surgical grade stainless steel. Once you've got nickel dermatitis, it's too late.

Q: How about fourteen-karat gold? It's perfectly safe, isn't it?

A: I wish I could answer yes, but unfortunately, quite a bit of fourteen-karat gold contains leachable nickel, that is, nickel which can be drawn out by sweat, water, detergents, and so forth. So to be safe, you should stick to stainless steel.

DERMALERT

Even fourteen-karat gold can contain nickel which can be drawn out by your body. To be safe, stick with surgical grade stainless steel for earring posts.

Q: I dab my earlobes and earring posts with alcohol and have never had one bit of trouble. Does alcohol help, really?

A: Probably. Isopropyl alcohol (common rubbing alcohol) is really quite a good antibacterial agent. It probably keeps the number of bacteria so low that the probability of an infection of the pierced ear tract is remote. But once the tract made by the piercing instrument is fully healed, such infections are extremely rare anyway. So it's probably wise to use alcohol for the first three weeks or so, until the holes are fully healed.

Moisturizers and Wrinkles

Q: Can moisturizer really prevent wrinkles?

A: Only sun avoidance prevents wrinkles. Moisturizers only soften the superficial skin a *little*, making it feel *slightly* better and more supple. The wrinkles just laugh at the stuff. You should also realize that some of the least expensive moisturizers anywhere, such as Complex-15 and Lubriderm, actually do a *better* job of moisturizing the skin without ill effects (such as acne cosmetica, allergies, and irritation) than the very expensive ones.

Food Facials

Q: I read a book on "kitchen cosmetics," in which people were told to put lime juice and vitamin E on the face. Is this really okay?

A: No! Lime juice is one of the most potent photosensitizers known. That means that, if you are exposed to even small amounts of sunlight, a fairly violent rash can occur. It's all right to *eat* limes, but never let the juice or rind come in contact with your skin.

You know already that we consider vitamin E to be off limits for the skin because of the propensity it has to cause topical skin allergy.

DERMALERT

Remember this equation: lime juice + sunlight = blistering skin rash!

Smoking—A Cause of Wrinkles?

Q: Does smoking affect a woman's skin?

A: Several years ago a study was published stating you could tell the side on which a woman held her cigarette while smoking by the severity of wrinkles on that side. The authors maintained that this may be due to squinting as smoke wafts by the eyes. They also considered the possibility that some noxious chemical might be causing the skin to wrinkle.

When researchers sought to reproduce the study, it was shown to be, for the most part, invalid. I can only say in my experience as a clinician seeing thousands of women for all sorts of skin problems, I think that smoking women *are* more severely and more coarsely wrinkled than the nonsmokers.

Hand Eczema—A Fistful of Problems

Q: Three years ago, my hands began to form blisters, and since then I have never had clear hands even once. The scaly areas and cuts are very painful, but I have learned to live with it to a degree by telling myself there is no cure.

My doctor says it is due to nerves and stress. Of my six brothers and sisters, five of them have been bothered with eczema, as was my mother. If there is anything you might know concerning my problem, I would be very grateful.

A: Oh, the pain of hand eczema! Millions of women know the trouble it can cause, and I thank you for sending in a question about the troubles it has caused you.

Eczema means red, scaly, easily irritated skin. We don't know the exact cause, but we do know it's *not* contagious. And, as you've stated, it does run in families.

In certain cases, eczema is a skin allergic reaction. Sometimes this can be tracked down with extensive patch testing, which will show contact allergy to one or more chemicals. These tests are done by applying the actual chemicals to the skin of the upper back. Occlusive patches and tape are used to maximize penetration so that they are more available to your immune systems: the skin's reactions can be thus discovered more easily.

The patches are applied on one day and are read two days later for signs of itching, redness, swelling, bumps, and blisters. The angrier the reaction, the more significant the test result. I've had several cashiers, for instance, who were quite violently allergic to nickel, and handling coins was causing their hand problem.

I encourage patients with hand eczema to bring in everything they've used on their skin, including lotions, cosmetics, cleaning agents, detergents, soaps, perfumes, and shampoos. Many patients with hand and arm eczema turn out to be violently allergic to their shampoos.

While we don't currently know the exact cause of hand eczema, we do know many of the aggravants. Hand eczema occurs much more frequently in housewives, bartenders, cocktail waitresses, assembly line workers, and others who have their hands frequently immersed in water.

Even though hand eczema is sometimes called *dyshidrosis*, which means "painful sweating," it has nothing at all to do with the sweat glands of the hands. The old-timers used to think that the tiny, deep-seated blisters under the hand skin were sweat glands "welling up with disease," but thorough biopsies have shown these to be completely unrelated to the sweat glands themselves. Dyshidrosis also frequently occurs of the feet.

Because of the bad drying effects of water on the hands, keep your hands out of water whenever possible.

DERMALERT

Water is the deadly enemy of hands with eczema.

How can you keep your hands dry when you must bathe your children, wash dishes, and do other household tasks? The best way is to buy three or four pairs of Dermal gloves and use these thin cotton gloves as liners under your regular rubber gloves. The reason for this is to always have a dry surface next to your hands. When one set of liners gets moist, either from splashing water into your gloves or from sweating, change liners. In this way, you'll keep a dry surface next to your sensitive hands all the time. If you can't get them at your local pharmacy, the address for the Dermal gloves is:

George Glove Company, Inc.
27 Haynes Avenue
Newark, New Jersey 07114

The next most common aggravant to hand eczema is soap. Try to avoid the antibacterial deodorant soaps. In general, they're too drying for hands that tend to get hand eczema. Also, those new liquid soaps in the sink-side dispensers are horribly drying. I suggest you use Dove, since it has recently been found (in two separate studies) to be the mildest soap. What about baby soap? It *is* a mild soap, but because it is assumed to be so much milder than other soaps, my patients tend to get into trouble with it because they use too much of it and because they use it too frequently. Stick with Dove—no one's ever found one milder.

Still, though, the best soap is the one which is never used! In fact, many dermatologists suggest that their patients use only three to five drops of Cetaphil lotion because of its tremendous mildness for eczematous hands. The lotion is applied, rubbed into a lather to cleanse the hands, and wiped off with a tissue, so that absolutely no water (other than that contained in the Cetaphil) ever touches the skin in the washing process.

Don't forget to rinse your hands well after each soap and water wash (if you absolutely *must* wash), and immediately thereafter apply a good moisturizing lotion such as Complex 15, Ultra Derm, Aquacare, Ultra Mide, or Carmol 10. These lotions allow you to maintain moisture in the skin of your hands by reapplying the natural skin oil you just removed.

While it goes without saying that harsh, irritating chemicals, such as solvents, turpentine, cutting oils, and detergents, should be kept miles from your delicate hands, you should know that vegetable juices like potato juice and onion juice will also greatly aggravate your hands.

For the present, there's no cure for hand eczema, but by following my advice you can keep your hands in the best shape possible at almost all times.

Once again, at the risk of breaking the bubble of those I prefer to call "psychodermatologists," I'll state again that nerves don't affect hand eczema one bit. Jerry, a lawyer friend of mine, has horrible hand eczema, even at some of the calmest times in his life. At other, more stressful times, of which he has plenty, Jerry gets no worse. So I've never been a very staunch believer in the mind's control over the skin. Altogether too many physicians are, however, and I think that's unfortunate for patients.

Q: I get a burning reaction on my hands from handling a lot of our "central Kentucky favorite," hot banana peppers, deep-fried right from my garden. What would be a relief and treatment for these?

A: This type of reaction is really not an allergy, but something called a *primary irritant reaction*. In an actual allergy, the rash is produced by the workings of a complicated system of immune factors inside the body. It would *not* happen to everybody who contacted the substance, just those whose immune systems were competent enough to recognize the substance as foreign.

However, in a primary irritant reaction, such as you get from those wonderful peppers, everyone would get the reaction by handling enough of the offending substance. The cure is either not to handle them or else to wear rubber gloves when you do.

There is one exception to this situation which may have to be investigated for you by an allergist or a dermatologist. This is when contact with the peppers or other substances or certain chemicals causes a hivelike reaction. This is called *contact urticaria syndrome*, and can be quite severe, even life-threatening. So if your hands swell and get very red on immediate contact with the peppers, see your physician right away. Incidentally, contact urticaria syndrome can happen with some of the oddest substances. One report concerned a little girl who swelled up every time her dog licked her. The dog's saliva activated the hivelike reaction.

Q: I have a lot of cracking and bleeding around the fingernails. What causes this, and is there a treatment? Is it caused by
a virus?

A: The cracking and bleeding around the fingernails sounds
like a variant of hand eczema which has occurred primarily in this
location on your hands. Some women get the reaction mainly in
the paronychial areas (the areas around the nail).

There are some other things to consider with the scaly paronychial areas, however. Women who use a lot of nail polish often
dry out the skin around their nails by using too much acetone
nail polish remover. I advise them to leave their polish on as long
as they can, or to completely stop using polish for a while. This,
plus a routine of heavy moisturization with a cream like Complex-
15, should help tremendously.

The Itchy Neck—Healing It for Good

Q: I've been told I've got neurodermatitis on the back of my
neck and scalp. What's neurodermatitis? Treatment?

A: Neurodermatitis is another one of those more or less psy-
chodermatological terms. The real name for this disease is *lichen
simplex chronicus,* a Latin term meaning "skin which thickens and
scales due to long-term scratching." It usually starts out as a minor
itching place on the back of the neck and scalp area. Scratching
the spot damages the skin a little, and it heals ever so slightly
thicker than before. That's because the skin's trying to protect
itself by thickening. As healing progresses, the itch fibers in the
skin are activated again by slight scar contraction in the damaged
area. The new itching causes more scratching, damage, thickening, healing, and itching, and so on, and on, and on!

This is the itch-scratch cycle, and it can continue incessantly
unless something happens to interrupt it. Usually, that something
is a cortisone gel, cream, or liquid, which can finally halt the
vicious itch-scratch cycle. Often we request that patients cut all
the white free edges off their nails, so that there's essentially
nothing there with which to scratch. We also ask patients to rub
a little medicine into the area with the *flat of their finger pad* every

time the spot itches. In this way, they do a modified "scratch" and apply their medicine at the same time. I've mentioned this technique previously in Chapter 4.

Cut Hosiery Bills—Cure Your Rough Heels

Q: I've got the worst damned heels in the country! They scale and crack constantly. I heard you mention a new medicine for this one time. Could you tell me more about it?

A: This problem, called *tylosis*, is a real annoyance to women, because the scaly areas on the heels can crack, bleed, and even run hosiery! While the problem occasionally has another cause, such as a fungus or an allergic contact dermatitis, it's more usually the result of severe dryness on the feet, especially the thick heel areas. There are even inherited cases which are quite extreme.

There are treatments for this problem, such as conventional moisturizers, soaks of various kinds, and over-the-counter medicines, but over the years, I've found a regimen which works better for my patients than any other I've ever tried. Ask your doctor for prescriptions for the two medicines, but I think you'll find it well worth the price of the office call. You may have to do this whole procedure only two to three times weekly to keep smoother feet.

It goes like this: Soak your feet in warm, clear tap water for about twenty to thirty minutes at night. Pat your feet dry, and apply a good layer of Keralyt gel (one of the prescription items) over the affected areas. Then cover each of your feet with a plastic bag, followed by a sock over the bag. You should *not* tape the bag down; just cover it with a sock. Leave this occlusive bandage on all night. Be careful not to slip with the plastic bags on your feet. Bags and carpets are a slippery combination.

In the morning, take off the bags, and wipe the sweat, dead skin cells, and remaining medicine off your feet. Then apply a good layer of Lac-Hydrin lotion (the other prescription medicine).

If you follow the above program regularly, I'm fairly certain that you won't have much of a problem with feet looking more like elephant hide than skin. Remember, you must see your doctor for this treatment, but it's worth it.

Genital Warts

Q: I have had vaginal warts for about three years and have had several different types of treatments by gynecologists and dermatologists. The treatments were painful and long-term. They have not spread recently, and my husband hasn't gotten any, but we're thinking of starting a family, and I'd like to know if the warts should be taken off before I have a baby. Is there any harm to the baby from these?

A: Viral warts grow like wildfire on some patients, absolutely defying the doctor's every attempt to annihilate them. In the vaginal area, because of the natural wetness, the nasty virus spreads with even greater alacrity.

Researchers have found that there are at least forty different types of wart virus. Some of these types smolder along for years, slowly decreasing the amount of infectious virus they secrete. Apparently, while they're becoming less and less infectious, they are also, unfortunately, becoming associated more and more with cancer in the vulvar area. That is, these long-term lesions are worrying researchers in the field that they may some day cause cancer. That's why, for the most part, we advise women to get these off as soon as practical. These facts aside, however, you wouldn't want your husband to show up with warts on his genitalia: so you really should have them removed.

More important, some virologists feel that laryngeal papillomas, small growths on the vocal cords, may be caused by contacting wart virus in the mother's birth canal during delivery. For that reason alone, vaginal warts should be treated.

Well, we've covered a lot of ground in this lengthy chapter. In Chapter 13, we'll talk about some very annoying problems that predominantly affect men.

13

His Skin

There was a guy in medical school who shook the entire first row
of seats while constantly scratching a groin itch. The annoyance
caused by this probably gave me my first hint that I was interested
in dermatology. Anyway, this fellow was dubbed "Itchy" by his
classmates, till he got to his dermatology rotation. There his at-
tending physician offered some help.

It turned out that the poor fellow had had "jock itch" for twelve
years! Imagine his surprise when a month of special antifungal
pills made his lifelong scourge vanish. But you know how nick-
names stick. Some of his classmates still call him Itchy.

In this section, I'm going to teach you everything you ever
wanted to know about some troublesome problems, like jock itch,
related predominantly to males.

Two-Foot-One-Hand Disease

Q: I came home from Vietnam with one hand and its nails in a pitiful state. It's so bad I've even been considering having my nails taken off. The hand is scaly and my nails are thick with crumbly stuff up under them all the time. I have this condition on the skin and nails of both my feet also. I heard you mention some internal medicine that might stop the fungus. What is this and will it help me?

A: Your description of the fungus affecting your hands and feet could be right out of a textbook! We call what you have "two-foot-one-hand disease," or, in medical terms, *tinea*. It is the result of a stubborn fungus which, like long strands of vegetable matter, actually grows into the upper layers of skin, where it multiplies. Sometimes, as in your case, it lasts for years and can affect the fingernails severely, causing them to be so thick that they are functionally unusable.

The great mystery is: Why does the fungus grow only on one hand? Frankly, we don't have the answer to what causes this strange condition. Researchers have tried to relate it to handedness, thinking that one hand would undergo different conditions than the other, but such theories appear to be invalid. Perhaps the immune system is responsible, but the answer is not yet in. Much more research is needed to adequately explain two-foot-one-hand disease.

The longest-lasting case I've ever seen was that of a 40-year-old farmer who showed up in my office a couple of years ago. He was explaining to me a problem of "diesel oil irritation" on his right hand. He had had it for twenty years! He showed me a fine, powdery scale on his right palm, which aroused my suspicion. When I asked him to show me his feet, both were *covered* with the classical thick scale of tinea pedis (foot fungus) infection.

DERMALERT

Fine, powdery scale on two feet and one hand is a fungus infection.

Worst of all, the fingernails on the affected hand and most of his toenails were as thick as horses' hoofs. I told him what he had, but he insisted it was just diesel oil irritation, caused by a spill of fuel onto his hand long ago. So I did what's called a KOH preparation on the scaly material to demonstrate the fungus. When I looked into the microscope, the scale contained so much fungus that I thought it would reach out and grab me!

I told him the good news. An oral antifungal pill called *griseofulvin* could probably heal his hand and feet over a period of time. Hands usually take six months or so, but toenails and feet, much more difficult areas to clear, can take as long as 1 to 1½ years. It takes twelve to eighteen months to grow a new toenail, but only six to nine months to grow a new fingernail.

Over the next few months, his hands began to clear for what I'm sure must have been the first time in his adult life. He's about the most grateful patient I've ever seen! He really never thought he'd have a smooth hand again.

Nail Fungus—Hard as Nails to Treat

Q: I have had a fungus infection under all my fingernails for over a year. It got better when I used a number of ointments, but it comes right back from time to time. Why don't the *topical* agents work?

A: The nail is made of a waterproof protein called *keratin*, which is specially built to protect the end of the digit and to keep chemicals, including antifungals *out*, not let them in. That makes the job of the pharmacologist, or drug designer, doubly hard, because, in a sense, the skin is working against its own cure.

The simple fact is that normal lotions which will kill a fungus in almost every other skin area will not touch those beneath the nail. That's why oral medicines, which get to the nail fungus from the inside, are needed.

Q: My father-in-law has a fungus which he's had in the toenails for over nineteen years. His toenails become quite thick, fibrous, and hard. Is there any way to get that thick stuff off the toe? It seems like it would heal better if we could. It hurts him to cut or clip them.

A: You're in luck! Or rather, your father-in-law's in luck. Over the last few years, a method has been developed for painless removal of diseased toenails. Called the beeswax-urea method, it was discovered in the Soviet Union, and was brought back to the United States by a prominent visiting dermatologist-professor. In our office we call it the "Russian formula" bandage.

The technique consists in the application of a paste made from beeswax and urea. These two ingredients soften the nail plate, but, remarkably, only where the plate has underlying disease, such as a fungus. The paste is plastered on the toenail, covered with a bandage, and left on for about seven to ten days, the bandage and paste are removed, and all the diseased nail is then trimmed off — painlessly! Patients can hardly believe how well it works. Sometimes, if the whole nail is diseased, it will come off completely and painlessly, all the way back to the nail fold (cuticle).

When the nail is removed, we usually put the patients on oral and topical antifungals, so that their risk of regrowing a fungus-laden nail is greatly lessened. Special tricks, such as filing the thick nail flat with an emery board so that it's paper thin, can also help greatly as the nail begins to reemerge.

Q: I have small blisters that are dark in color on the bottom of my right foot. There are none on the left. When they heal, the skin turns almost white in color and peels off very easily. Is this a fungus?

A: A professor in my residency had a favorite saying: A blister on the foot is fungus until proved otherwise. And he's absolutely right. Tiny, deep-seated blisters on the feet most often are fungus. It's really very easy to prove this when your doctor scrapes the top off one or more of the blisters. He or she can look at this material in the KOH preparation and confirm fungus in minutes.

DERMALERT

Blisters on the feet are a reliable indicator of foot fungus.

Of course, there really are a lot of other conditions which can cause blisters on the feet, but by far the most common one is foot fungus.

Jock Itch

Q: What causes jock itch?

A: *Jock itch* is a catchall term for over three different types of groin rash. The major one is tinea cruris, or fungus of the groin. It's usually a red rash seen in teens and older patients, almost always men. *Usually*, a fairly distinct reddish border is seen with tinea cruris. The border may be slightly raised, or swollen, and tends to be somewhat uneven in its outline. It rarely, if ever, crosses the crural fold. That's the fold where the legs attach to the groin. In other words, it almost never strikes the scrotum. It's treated with the medicines we are discussing for the other fungi, such as ringworm and foot fungus. It's fairly easy to clear up, but it can come back quite easily if the feet are infected with a fungus. Have them checked too, and treated if necessary.

However, moniliasis, a yeast infection quite common in men, does cross the crural fold onto the scrotum quite often. When there's a rash of moniliasis on the upper inner thighs, it's usually a spotty redness with what's known as *satellite papules*, or tiny, distinct bumps around the edges. These are usually separate from the main body of the groin rash. It's treated with antiyeast medicines such as Mycelex, Lotrimin, Monistat, Loprox, and Spectazole. Sometimes an older, but very effective, medicine, Fungizone, is used. All these medicines are obtained only through prescription.

The third common infectious cause of jock itch is erythrasma. This is an infection caused by a bacterium called *Proprionibacterium minutissimum*. The most peculiar fact about this organism is that it secretes a chemical which glows coral red in the presence of a black light called a Wood's light, and that's the way dermatologists make the diagnosis. It's commonly treated with topical and internal antibiotics, which kill off the infecting bacteria quite rapidly.

There are at least three different infectious types of jock itch. It's not always fungus.

A Fungus Running Around in Circles

Q: Is jock itch the same as ringworm? How is it spread? Where's the worm?

A: Yes, it's really ringworm of the groin. First, there's *no* worm in ringworm. But the circular lesions, or spots, of this fungus certainly give one the impression that there might be. The term may have been around for over 500 years, and was probably used to describe not only the ringlike lesions of skin fungus, but also psoriasis, eczema, syphilis, and many other diseases through the centuries.

Why does it spread in a circle? No one knows. It may very well have something to do with the immune system, but as yet we're not smart enough to figure it out. Maybe each individual cell the fungus attacks acquires immunity to it, allowing the fungus to spread in only one direction—outward. This results in the formation of a circle as it progresses.

We do know it's contagious, however. Ringworm of the scalp, for instance, used to be an almost occupational disease of moviegoers. The backs of old-time theater seats were chock full of the fungus, and many unlucky kids caught "the tetter" from leaning their heads back to watch the show.

Treatment of tinea corporis (ringworm) is much the same as treatment of the other fungi we've discussed, but the time needed to resolve it is usually vastly less. Often a month of internal treatment will be enough. Obviously, there is no worm.

It's the Pits!

Q: My problem is unbelievable. I don't have jock itch; I've got "pits itch." My armpits itch almost constantly, and the armpit hairs are full of a yellow-gray coating which I can't remove. I think my skin's okay; it's the *hairs* that need help. Help, the crud's got me!

A: You've probably got a condition called *trichomycosis axillaris*. In this disease, bacteria adhere to the hairs but not the skin. The hairs stick together and become a real nuisance. No one knows exactly why it strikes predominantly the armpits. Of course women who shave their underarms regularly don't have much problem with trichomycosis axillaris.

Treatment, as you may have guessed, is simple. Shave your underarms. If you don't like that prospect, you can get various topical antibiotics from your doctor, or use a 1% formalin lotion, which could be made up by your pharmacist.

Penile Warts

Q: I have large warts on my penis. One of them is really huge, measuring about an inch across! Will they eventually fall off? Any dangers to them? How do you treat them?

A: Warts on the genitals are called *venereal warts*. In every single case, because of their contagious nature, they. should be treated. It's not easy, and even painful at times, but if you value protecting your sex contacts from them, have your skin doctor treat them.

The treatments for warts include podophyllin, electrocautery, cryosurgery, conventional surgery, and laser surgery. Podophyllin is a plant resin which irritates the warts off your skin — if you're lucky! Occasionally it causes so much irritation that cortisone medications are necessary to cool down the area. This medicine is dangerous, from this standpoint, and should *never* be dispensed by prescription for the patient's use. It's always put on in the doctor's office. The doctor will give you very specific instructions on washing it off in four to eight hours. Do this *exactly* as your doctor instructs.

Electrocautery is mentioned only to condemn it. Burning off warts went out with the ancients, and certainly should not be used on one of the most important and tender areas of the body.

Cryosurgery (freezing the wart off with liquid nitrogen) is my favorite choice for genital warts. It makes a small scab out of the wart, which will drop off in a week or two. Of course, the areas should be checked as often as possible to guard against recurrences. Recurrent small warts should be refrozen as soon as you notice them. This treatment stings a bit but is very effective.

Conventional scalpel removal of warts is usually avoided because of scarring.

Laser treatment of warts is now becoming popular because of the great ability of the laser light to virtually vaporize tissue on contact. You'll hear a lot more about this technique in the future. I've referred many cases of extremely large warts to expert laser surgeons, and the results have been marvelous.

Your large wart gives me cause for concern, because certain large warts can have skin cancer in their bases. Any large wart, therefore, should be treated as soon as possible, and if it is recurrent, a biopsy should be performed to check for this disease.

Beards and Shaving

Q: What can a person do to make his beard grow thicker in the sparse areas? I'm in my late teens, and it's just not filling out the way I'd like it to.

A: Your beard growth is determined by your individual set of genes. They tell it when to start and where to grow. And unless you've already had hair in the areas of which you speak, and it's *decreased* there now, there's not much you can do about making it grow where it doesn't want to. Sorry. But take a close look at your uncles on both sides of your family and at your dad. You'll get some idea of what your permanent beard pattern will be.

Q: Does shaving stimulate hair growth?

A: No. Read Chapter 10 for further information and the reasons why not.

Q: What are the dangers in shaving over a mole or birthmark on my face?

A: If the mole sticks out a distance from the skin, the obvious hazard is cutting it recurrently. Does this cause cancer? Probably not, but it can cause confusion, in that any redness could be interpreted as a precancerous or frankly cancerous change by your physician. If that happens, then he or she is likely to recommend the complete removal of the mole.

If it sticks up above the surface, therefore, I'd have my skin doctor see if it would be best to take it off via the shave biopsy technique, to lessen the effect of shaving over it.

DERMALERT

If a mole is constantly traumatized, it should be removed, not because the trauma causes cancer but because it causes confusion and concern.

Remember, however, that if, as I mentioned in Chapter 3, a dark mole has been present ever since birth, most dermatologists would advise removal of it anyway.

Tattoos

Q: My husband has a three-inch tattoo (a product of his youth) on the back of his arm. He was advised earlier that surgical removal would leave a large scar and draw the tissue on the back of the arm too tight.

I read somewhere that lasers are being used for this problem. Are you familiar with such a procedure? Is there someone in our area that my husband could consult?

A: Lasers may well be the best way to remove this large tattoo. You've heard me talk about lasers in dermatology before, and I'd certainly look into finding a laser specialist for a consultation. If you're looking for a reputable specialist who does a certain medical procedure in your area, always be sure to call the local medical society and the local university's department of dermatology if there's one nearby. One or the other should be able to refer you. If not, you may call the American Academy of Dermatology at 312-869-3954, or write them at:

The American Academy of Dermatology
820 Davis Street
P.O. Box 271
Evanston, Illinois 60201

Don't expect a "no-scar result," however, with any means of tattoo removal. That pigment is deep within the dermis, or second layer of the skin, and it's tough to get out. The laser's light is so powerful that when it strikes the pigment in the area the pigment is vaporized into smoke immediately. But the heat of the procedure does induce some scarring, just as would a third-degree burn in the same area.

Hopefully, with this information about "his skin" you'll be able to live more comfortably without many of the problems which predominantly affect males. Some are difficult and/or painful to treat, but how much better life is without them!

In my experience, men are much more reluctant than women to have annoying skin problems treated. Sadly, this often leads to years of suffering for lack of a little proper dermatologic treatment. It's my hope that this chapter for men will encourage those with problems to seek treatment.

14

Black Skin—Some Good News and Some Bad News

Black skin is a magnificent organ which contains its own sun protection, the pigment melanin. This brownish-black pigment is produced in a host of tiny pigment cells called melanocytes lying in an almost unbroken layer along the bottom cell layer of the epidermis. In some areas there are virtually thousands per square centimeter. The pigment they produce is an incredible sunshield! It's so effective, in fact, that sun-induced skin cancer is extraordinarily rare among blacks, and wrinkling is greatly retarded too.

Amazingly, there are about the same number of pigment-producing melanocytes in black and in white skin. In blacks, however, the melanocytes crank out more melanin and melanin of different types than that secreted by Caucasians.

Melanocytes are very responsive cells. Sunlight and all kinds of other injuries can make them turn on like little factories to crank out mountains of pigment when it's needed (and, as we shall see, sometimes when it's not!).

So the good news is that black skin is resistant to skin cancer. It's also slightly less likely to contract contact allergy. What about oriental-type skin? In Orientals, the actual molecular *type* of melanin and the distribution of the pigment are different. Dr. Ken Hashimoto, Chairman of Dermatology at Wayne State University, says that major surveys have been done in the Japanese population. "Orientals have very rare basal cell carcinomas and rare premalignant actinic keratoses (sunspots). In this sense, oriental skin is more resistant to skin cancer than is Caucasian skin, but somewhat less resistant to skin cancer than black skin."

Renowned dermatologist Ernst Epstein goes even further in stating that he cannot remember (in his extensive experience) ever seeing a melanoma in an oriental patient! He is quick to caution that he is sure they occur, but in his practice, he's not seen them.

Black skin, however, has some special problems. Among those problems more prevalent in blacks is a serious one called razor dermatitis.

Beard Bumps (Razor Dermatitis)

Q: My 19-year-old son has a problem with shaving in the neck area. He can't use shaving preparations because they irritate his skin. He tried an electric razor but the problem just goes on. Is there a razor which would be worth a try?

A: Your son appears to have the very annoying condition called *pseudofolliculitis barbae*, or PFB. PFB (razor dermatitis or razor bumps) is an inflammation or irritation produced where curly beard hairs repenetrate the facial and neck skin, causing inflammation or soreness. Note that the irritation is not where the hairs come *out* of the skin, but at the site of *repenetration*. That's why it's called *pseudo-*, or *false*, folliculitis. While this occurs very commonly in blacks, some curly-haired whites also have the problem.

Shaving is the definitive *cause* of PFB, so that stopping shaving brings about a very rapid improvement. The worst thing that patients can do is to continue shaving.

We have known for a long time that the definitive cure for PFB is growing a beard. While the beard is coming out we encourage the men to flip out these small, repenetrating hairs (called "bucket handles") from the skin where they are growing back in.

This can be done with a toothpick, and allows the beard to grow without curling hairs up inside the skin.

If circumstances prohibit the growing of a beard, which is often the case for people in business and in the military, we ask patients to wash the facial area with a Buf-Puf and a mild soap. Then the skin is well dried and various medications can be applied. These include topical antibiotics and antiacne preparations such as vitamin A acid (Retin-A) and benzoyl peroxide. A word should also be said about the type of razor used. The worst of all possible razors is the double-track razor. With this twin-bladed razor, the first blade cuts off the hair and the second blade often slices off a small bump of skin below the hair. This causes secondary infection, scarring, and facilitates repenetration of the hair back into the skin.

DERMALERT

Razor bumps are often repenetrating hairs. Shaving, especially with a twin-bladed razor, makes them worse!

An electric razor is still the least traumatic for the skin, if your son decides he cannot tolerate a beard. If he uses an electric razor, a light oil preshave, such as Williams' 'Lectric Shave, may be used so that the surface of the razor will glide more easily.

Keloids—Scars Gone Wild

Q: Three years ago I had a modified mastectomy, and about four inches of the scar is now a very tender keloid. My surgeon has never recommended anything to put on it. I've used cocoa butter and various body lotions, but it still remains very tender. Is there anything for this type of scar tissue?

A: Keloids are very common in blacks, less common in olive-skinned people, and rare in Caucasians. Minor keloids are called *hypertrophic* (overgrown) scars, but keloids themselves go further than just simple enlargement. They grow out of and away from their natural boundaries, and extend to normal skin.

In blacks, they start out as a reddish scar which swells up above the surrounding skin and gets progressively harder. As time passes, they acquire a brownish pigmentation, and then usually darken intensely to a skin tone several shades deeper than the usual skin color for the area.

Although surgical wounds are the most common sites where keloids develop, they do occur in many other types of injury such as acne lesions, cuts, scrapes, and burns.

You don't mention whether you or your family are prone to forming these scars. This would have been helpful to know before your surgery, so that some precautions could have been taken. For instance, many doctors will anesthetize the surgical site with a numbing medicine mixed with cortisone, so that it's less likely to heal with a big scar.

Pierced ears account for the majority of keloids in my practice, and they're one of the biggest headaches to get rid of too. Of course, pierced ears are the rage in our society, so it's unlikely that I could convince people not to have the piercing procedure done, but black women deserve a special note of caution. This operation can cause keloids to form regardless of *who* does the piercing. And once the keloid forms, it's very difficult, if not impossible, to get rid of it.

Most ear piercing is done in a department store by nonmedical personnel. That means that you may have problems with infection and nickel allergy, as well as scarring. Were this not so, do you think they'd make you sign that long form prior to your piercing operation? I don't stand alone when I say that surgery should only be done by surgeons. That means that laypersons, no matter what training they have, are unlikely to be able to adequately advise you on the possible complications of the procedure.

Unfortunately, I've seen ear keloids as big as a walnut on black patients. Ordinarily, with a lump or bump somewhere, you'd just expect the surgeon to excise the lesion. In keloids, however, that often results in the regrowth of the lesion to an even bigger size! Treatment often involves the use of cortisone injections, and also radiation therapy to control subsequent scarring. Sometimes, even with these treatments, the keloids *still* come back bigger than they were originally. You can see that keloids are not an easy problem.

Q: Can anything be done for the itching in keloids?

A: The cortisone injections often clear up the itching in a few days. Topical cortisone creams also help itching, but you should be careful to apply the medicine *only* to the keloid to prevent the medicine from thinning the skin around it.

Q: I am 33 years old and have had to live with a long scar for a gallbladder operation since I was 20. This is very embarrassing especially during swimming season. Should I have this scar revised by a plastic surgeon, and if so, whom should I talk to about it?

A: Your gallbladder scar will have all the problems I've mentioned about the other forms of keloids, with one notable additional problem. Gallbladder scars often turn out badly because there is so much tension on that area of the abdominal skin that they stretch and spread very easily. Revision by a plastic surgeon engenders the same risks as revision of the scars on the earlobes caused by piercing. However, you should consult your local plastic surgeon. He or she will tell you, after an examination and after taking your history, whether or not surgery would result in a successful revision of the scar.

Cornrow Hair Loss

Q: My daughter likes to cornrow her hair, but now, after several years of tight braids, I don't think she's got as much hair, especially in the areas between the rows. Am I using the wrong kind of shampoo for her?

A: We see all too much of this problem. The condition is called *traction alopecia*. It's a real hazard for blacks who desire to have the new plaited hairstyles, especially the very fine braids, because these braids exert fantastic traction—or pulling stresses—on the scalp hairs.

With this chronic pulling of the hairs, scarring is induced deep down in the follicle where the hair is made. This results in the gradual obliteration of the active hair-growing apparatus, and with it, permanent hair loss. This is the same kind of process that results in loss of hair in nurses who pin on their caps so tightly that they begin to lose hair over the years.

Traction alopecia can be a true disaster if it's not recognized and stopped quickly. Braiding of the hair does *not* have to stop altogether, but at least the tension on the base of the hairs where they are attached to the scalp should be lessened. Start braiding very loosely so that almost no tension is put on the scalp skin. Ask your daughter to *tell* you when and if it begins to feel tight. Often the child can tell the tightness a lot better than the mother. Cornrowing is okay, but do it right and avoid possible permanent hair loss.

Darker Spots

Q: Every time I hurt my skin, whether it's a scratch, a scrape, or just an irritated place, my natural brown skin tone there gets much darker. Why does it do that, and how can it be fixed?

A: Remember the tiny color cells, or melanocytes, that we talked about at the start of this chapter? These diminutive pigment factories are most efficient producers of brown pigment, and usually they do it in a very regular, controlled fashion. This gives the skin an even brownish to black coloration. However, any physical trauma can greatly stimulate the output of melanin, causing the skin to darken drastically in just a matter of days.

There are two components to this pigment darkening—an epidermal, or surface, darkening and a dermal, or deeper, darkening. The epidermal type of pigment will usually resolve with time. The dermal deposits, however, are another story. They are not likely to lighten to normal skin tone very quickly, if at all. Sometimes it takes years for this type of stain to lighten significantly. In rare cases, the spots are permanent, just like tattoos.

Hypermelanosis, as the spots of extra dark pigment are called, is best treated by "tincture of time" therapy. That is, most dermatologists would choose to wait for the spots to improve naturally before resorting to a pigment lightener. Among the available lighteners is Melanex, which we've previously discussed in the chapter dealing with melasma, the mask of pregnancy. It's a prescription drug available only through your doctor.

Of critical importance is halting or ameliorating whatever caused the darkening in the first place. I'll give you an example. Sylvia, a black patient with acne, had discovered that a loofah sponge made her facial skin feel soft and smooth. She liked the feel of it so much that she started using her loofah three or four times a day! She forgot how harsh these scrubbers are, and soon noticed some pigment darkening on her face which she tried even harder to scrub away. Sylvia realized too late that the dark spots, now huge brown-black triangles on her face, were actually *caused* by the scrubbing process!

I stopped Sylvia's use of the loofah, and put her on antibiotics for her acne. She began to clear quite rapidly, but the total time to achieve normal skin color was over ten months. So if you have black skin, be careful with it. It'll pigment at the slightest provocation.

15

Fingernails—Proper Care of Our "First Tools"

One cool summer morning, the first cavedweller was bitten by the first flea. The cavedweller instinctively scratched the itchy wound with a fingernail and unwittingly became the first human user of a tool in the world's history.

Actually, this story isn't as farfetched as it sounds, for our nails are truly responsible for our ability to manipulate fine objects. This function still persists, naturally—just watch someone trying to remove an adhesive bandage, or separate a sticky label from its backing, or perform any of a thousand other daily functions for which we use our nails, and you'll realize their importance.

But with civilization came another function of fingernails. They are now considered just as important for their decorative function. Everyone wants good-looking nails, and this chapter will tell you the up-to-date secrets to maintaining these important skin appendages in their best shape.

Fingernails Have R-R-Ridges

Q: How about ridges on the fingernails? I'd like to know what causes them, and what I can do about them?

A: Fingernail ridges have a whole set of different causes. Chief among these is hand eczema, which we've discussed in Chapter 12. You see, the nails are made deep under the nail fold (cuticle) and then grow out slowly to appear as what we know as nail plate, the hard part of the nail. If any inflammation or irritation occurs around the nail fold area, it quite easily disturbs the growth pattern of the nail plate, producing a ridge.

The second leading cause of fingernail ridging is manipulation of the cuticle. Cuticle means "little skin," and as a tiny patch of normal skin, it takes care of itself completely, *needing absolutely no help from us.* Certainly, a small amount of skin temporarily hangs onto and drifts out onto the nail plate from time to time, but that was meant to be there as a protection for the delicate tissues below which are actively engaged in making the nail plate. Vigorous pushing back of the cuticles, therefore, will cause ridging in almost everyone.

Several years ago, a company was distributing a new nail product. They sent crews to the largest and best department stores in the land to give demonstrations. The product was basically an extremely refined polishing system designed to remove surface lines and ridges from the nails. It did this so well that customers did not even have to wear nail polish, and they still looked as if they were wearing an ultrasmooth coat of clear polish at the time.

Needless to say, I was impressed. My wife and I caught up with them one spring day in a department store in Atlanta, and decided to try the stuff. She loved it, and coaxed me into letting them try one of my nails, so that I could recommend it to my patients. When the demonstrator heard that, she was determined to give me a good impression of the system, so she really put some pressure into the polishing steps. There were several steps, and when she finished, my thumbnail shone like the sun! I was ecstatic that I had made this wonderful discovery, and couldn't wait to get back to my residency in Augusta to tell everyone what I had found. We were, of course, always looking for a magical way to smooth out rough nails for our patients with psoriasis, eczema, and fungus problems.

We residents were recommending the stuff almost daily for a couple of weeks, till I noticed something strange happening to my demonstration nail. I was growing a huge, deep ridge out from under my cuticle. Aghast, we all waited for our patients to come back with the same ridges, and sure enough, they began to complain of this over the next several weeks. They all grew out normal nails again, but we surely had a group of worried residents for a while.

So you can see the effects of any pushing or trauma on the cuticle area. Treat these tender areas gently, and they'll continue to make you a smooth nail plate. Vigorous pushing back of the cuticles can cause deep ridges in the nails. Cuticles are normal. Leave them alone. Vigorous buffing also ridges nails. Beware!

Q: What are the other causes of ridges in the nails?

A: Psoriasis and other diseases, such as thyroid abnormalities, can also cause ridging of the nails. Your dermatologist can investigate these further. Sometimes if the underlying cause is corrected, the nails get better.

Q: Why would a middle-aged lady have really severe surface ridges on the toenail, particularly the large toe.

A: Ridges have many causes, but ridges on the toenails, and *not* simultaneously on the fingernails, suggest trauma as a main cause. That is, it's very possible that something you're doing to your toenails could be causing them. How about tight footwear? That's one of the chief causes of the large toenail ridges. Are you in an occupation where things often drop on your feet? Had any injuries over the last few months which might be showing up now? Remember that toenails only grow about two millimeters per month, so an injury could be two months old or so before you'd even *see* it!

I remember dropping a table knife on my great toe about five years ago, and the ridge and bruise didn't grow out and show up for weeks. Try to search your memory for injuries; it may produce some satisfying results.

Have Your Nails Gone Schiz?

Q: In the last year my nails have split back in layers. I have never had trouble with my nails before, and could always grow them to a nice length. Now, as soon as they get past the end of the finger, they split. I work in a bank and use finger moistening products to help in counting the money, and I wonder if this could cause it? Is there a simple way to prevent this?

A: This problem is one we all have to some degree, called *onychoschizia* (splitting of the nails). It's perhaps the most common complaint we hear about nails. The causes are vague, to say the least. One of the world's leading nail experts, Dr. Nardo Zaias, says, in his book, *The Nail in Health and Disease*, SP Medical & Scientific Books, 1980, "This layering of the nail plate is not an uncommon abnormality. *Absolutely nothing is known about it!*" (Italics and exclamation, mine.)

In practice, however, there are some things which do seem to aggravate onychoschizia. My patients get worse with this condition when they are in water frequently. Also, as with other nail problems, using polish remover frequently worsens it. And I would certainly eliminate the moistening agent for a while to see if you get better. I also think most of my patients do better if they keep their nails polished all the time. Agents such as Hard as Nails may help, too. Try not to be too conscientious about removing all the polish for what could be just a minor touch-up.

There are a few other secrets you should know about keeping your nails in good shape. Throw away your nail clipper, and get a sharp, new one every three months. Clip your nails only when they're wet (say, after a shower or bath). After you clip your nails, file them gently with a fresh emery board. Use a "down-and-away" motion from front to back on the nail edge.

And if you do still have a problem with nail splitting, use a heavy moisturizer containing phospholipids, urea, or lactic acid to soften your nails. If you use such lotions frequently, you may not have further problems with splitting.

Q: I have nails that keep splitting. I asked my doctor about it and he said, "Eat lots of gelatin," which I do. Does gelatin really cure the problem?

A: Being a scientist, I cringe when I hear someone utter that dermatologic falsehood. It's equivalent to the tribe of headhunters who reportedly said that if you wanted to be as brave as someone else, you must eat his heart, and so forth. If you want to have the best fingernails, must you eat modified fingernails (gelatin is ground-up horses' hoofs)? How disgusting. And it doesn't work. The protein provided by gelatin is constantly made available to your nail-making apparatus anyway. So give up the gelatin habit. One nail expert thinks it may even do more good to *soak* your nails in gelatin than to drink the stuff!

DERMALERT

Gelatin does nothing for nail splitting (onychoschizia).

Q: How about calcium to harden the nails?

A: It's completely useless. Calcium is used to make bones and teeth hard as nails, not vice versa!

Q: I, like most of my friends, wear artificial fingernails. The glue that comes with the nails will not keep them on, so we all discovered three or four years ago that Super Glue will keep them on at least a week. I, for one, wear them all the time, since I have bad nails with ridges and indentations. Is there any harm in this practice?

A: Did you give any thought to the possibility that your ridges are *caused* by the nails you're gluing on all the time? It's possible. I've got one patient who went to a salon where they use the cyanoacrylate glue of which you speak. She has become so allergic to this substance that her nails look worse than ever, and the cracking and irritation get so bad sometimes that she needs to get oral cortisone to shut down this horrible process. Still, she persists in using them occasionally. I guess she thinks that someday she'll lose her allergy to them, but that'll never happen.

DERMALERT

The glues used to anchor artificial nails, or to build them up, can cause allergies under and around the nails and may even cause loss of the nails.

Nail Dots and White Lies

Q: A long time ago, I had a lot of white spots on my fingernails, and someone told me that this was a lack of zinc. I took
some zinc and it seemed to help! Why don't you tell everyone to
do this?

A: Been telling white lies lately? That's where the little white
dots are supposed to come from, you know, at least according to
the old wives' tale. Actually, they come from minor nicks and
blows to the fingernails, causing a tiny dot of abnormal growth.
So no matter what you take, you will still get these spots if your
nails are hit from time to time. Zinc's useless for this purpose.

Realize that your nails are specialized organs of the skin. A
little regular maintenance of these delicate, useful, and beautiful
tools will keep them in shape for a lifetime.

16

Beating Psoriasis—How to Live Without Leaving a Trail of Scales

"Joe," said our department chairman on my first day on the dermatology rotation, "today you'll learn the cardinal sign of psoriasis. Somewhere in this clinic, there's a severe psoriatic. I want you to find him."

"Sure," I said naively, "no problem. Just let me look through these charts in the wall rack, and I'll find him in a minute."

"Whoa!" he exclaimed. "No charts; just stand right here and find him."

"Hmmm," I mumbled, with sweat now forming on my palms. "I'm afraid I haven't had my x-ray vision tuned up lately."

"Look around, doctor, the clues are here!"

I glanced down the long hallway leading to our exam rooms. All the doors were closed, and except for the unswept carpet, nothing was ... unswept carpet? *Unswept carpet*! That was it! Leading all the way down the hall was a long trail of branlike scales tracking right into room 12.

"Room 12?" I asked, with somewhat less than impressive confidence.

"Absolutely," the chief asserted. "That patient drops enough scale each day to enable you to track him anywhere! Now go see him firsthand. It's Mr. Williams, one of our chronic psoriatics."

Although not every psoriatic is as scaly as poor Mr. Williams, tremendous scaling can occur if psoriasis gets out of hand. The chairman's "find the psoriatic" lesson taught me about the torment of this dreadful disease. Let's consider some of the many questions on the minds of psoriatics.

Scales on Your Perfect Suit

Q: I have had psoriasis for a couple of years. Doctors give me the impression that this is something I'm always going to have. I've never gotten any better. What can I do?

A: First, you should not feel alone. The "heartbreak of psoriasis" strikes 1 to 5 percent of all of us. Virtually everyone has seen someone with it. In ancient times psoriasis was often confused with leprosy so that psoriasis victims tended to live the lives of outcasts. The rare tendency for psoriasis to undergo spontaneous remission may even account for some of the "miracle cures" in early religious history.

Scaling and redness are the hallmark of the disease. A quick look at the exact skin defect in psoriasis explains why. In normal skin the epidermis remakes itself from top to bottom about every thirty days. Ordinarily, the dead skin is constantly being sloughed off in an orderly fashion from the uppermost layer, the stratum corneum.

Imagine a perfectly fitting suit, renewing itself constantly and never wearing out. Skincredible! But in psoriasis lesions, called *plaques*, the skin speeds up its own replacement, so that its entire thickness is reproduced every *three* days. Ten times as fast as normal skin. No wonder it scales!

DERMALERT

Psoriasis spots scale because the skin of the spots remakes itself *ten times* as fast as normal skin.

The scaling of psoriasis is usually worst on the knees, elbows, genitalia, scalp, and between the buttocks. It is often a thick, whitish scale which early dermatologists called an "asbestos" or "silvery" scale because of its flaky, whitish-gray texture.

Often, the fingernails have small indentations or dot-sized dimples in the nail plates called *pits*. While occasional pits are normal, an increased number of pits, even ridges, due to lines of pits across the nail, may mean you've got the disease.

DERMALERT

> If your fingernails have tiny pits or dimples in the
> nail plates, you could have psoriasis.

Occasionally the scaling spreads from localized areas to the usually normal areas of the skin. Sometimes it covers the entire body, resulting in a condition called *exfoliative dermatitis*, which means "shedding of the skin." It can be a life-threatening problem, even involving heart failure. This happens when the severe inflammation of psoriasis causes the superficial skin blood vessels to open up wide. This massive dilatation of the miles and miles of skin blood vessels causes the effective blood volume of the body to decrease. Then the heart pumps even harder to try to supply the internal organs with blood, and eventually wears itself out. This is one of the few times that psoriasis can be fatal.

Patients with exfoliative dermatitis feel cold too, because all the wide-open blood vessels conduct the vital heat of the body to the surface. That's why these patients often shiver, even in the heat of summer. Remember, red skin in a psoriatic can indicate the presence of exfoliative dermatitis, a true dermatologic emergency. If this happens, see your doctor immediately!

Contagious—Never!

Q: For God's sake, tell me about it but don't make me touch it! Won't I catch something?

A: Along with the original "leprosy" fallacy about psoriasis, there are many other fallacies which should be dispelled. Psoriasis is not contagious. It's not an infection. Psoriatics are not unclean. As a matter of fact, one chief of dermatology at a large medical center illustrates this quite graphically to his new residents. He makes a bold point of his immediate warm handshake with even the scaliest of psoriatic patients, signaling with a quick commanding glance that the physicians-in-training should jump to follow his lead.

In fact, you can catch virtually *nothing* from an inflicted psoriatic. So if you know a psoriatic, or if you have the disease, stop worrying about catching it or spreading it to others. It may make a miserable disease a little more tolerable for the victim.

Genes Will Tell

Q: But how did I get psoriasis? I'm not allergic to *anything!*

A: Psoriasis is not an allergy, nor is it a problem primarily caused by "nerves" or emotions, although stress does seem to play a sizable role, as I'll mention when I talk about treatment.

Q: My dad has it, and my son has it too. Am I going to get it?

A: Unfortunately, there is *one* way in which the disease can be passed on—through inheritance. Almost 80 percent of my psoriatic patients have an affected relative. But there's no way to predict whether *you* will pass on the disease to *your* offspring. On the other hand, some psoriatics are known to have no relatives with the disease.

DERMALERT

Eighty percent of psoriatics have an afflicted relative, indicating that the disease is one of genetic transmission.

Long ago I learned firsthand about the hereditary nature of psoriasis when a biologist friend named Rob brought in his 6-year-old daughter. She had reddish scaly spots on her chest and some minor scaling on her elbows. Although I considered psoriasis in the diagnostic list, the December weather led me to dub her problem xerotic eczema (dry irritated skin patches) commonly seen in winter.

But when they returned three weeks later with new spots, her knees also had small patches with thick, whitish scale. A thorough check of her fingernails revealed numerous tiny pits, confirming psoriasis. Thorough questioning about relatives revealed no trace of the disease.

You can imagine my dismay almost a year later, when Rob brought in his second child, a tiny towhead named Darren, with scaly ears and scalp. I ever so cautiously dubbed this seborrheic dermatitis, an inflamed itchy dandruff condition, but I was really hoping against hope that it, too, wasn't psoriasis. I raised the possibility with Rob that Darren had psoriasis, but I hesitated to alarm him unduly unless the signs and symptoms worsened. Unfortunately, Darren's ears developed the thick, reddish scaly plaques which heralded the onset of the disease.

Not until two years later did I discover how important inheritance was to Rob's kids. Our office air conditioning was under repair on the hot summer day when he brought the kids in for a follow-up visit. Rob was in his shirt sleeves when I entered the room, and as I often do I shook his hand and gave him my usual friendly grip on the right arm and elbow with my left hand. As my fingers touched a scaly spot near his elbow, my friendly greeting turned to concern. I rotated his arm, stared at his psoriasis patch, and moaned a disappointed, "Not you too!" At last we knew the inheritance pathway of his kids' disease. Rob said he had had small "rough patches" on and off for years, but never related it to the kids' psoriasis.

Nutrition and Psoriasis

Q: Two members of our family with psoriasis have been taking special vitamins and they seem to have helped. I am convinced that nutrition is the key; how about you?

A: A bewildering amount of psoriasis research has been done

on its relationship to nutrition. In fact, basic research adds a new
and innovative treatment approach every few years. Unfortunately, nutritional therapy and vitamin supplements are not among
the ones that work. Long ago, proponents of the "turkey diet"
for psoriasis found that the only thing it cured was the anemic
wallets of the turkey producers. And I am sure that most of the
psoriatics who tried it thought that it was indeed a "fowl" diet!
But their psoriasis remained unchanged. Diet therapy is worthless
as a cure for psoriasis.

There are no magic vitamin cures for psoriasis. In fact, there
is one vitamin which can actually be harmful if applied topically—
vitamin E. As I've mentioned in an earlier chapter, topically applied vitamin E can cause a violent allergic sensitivity in the skin.
This was discovered years ago when vitamin E was introduced
in every form imaginable, from oils to deodorants to soaps. That's
when our offices filled with victims of contact allergy to vitamin E.

DERMALERT

Vitamin E is a topical contact sensitizer which can
cause a very itchy, poison ivy-like rash. So take it by
mouth if you must, where it does no harm, but do
not apply it to your skin.

Treating the "Heartbreak"

Q: Well, tell me about something that *does* work, then.

A: The most widely accepted treatment is the use of potent
topical cortisone creams and ointments applied frequently to the
skin lesions. They work by decreasing blood flow to the psoriasis
spots, a process called *vasoconstriction*. This process also decreases
redness, skin turnover rate, and therefore the thick scales of the
disease.

Q: I've had psoriasis for years on my lower legs. Are there
any soaps or lotions that help?

A: The lower legs are a tough nut to crack in psoriasis. The
lesions here are more stubborn than anywhere else on the body.
And soaps don't help. They usually dry, sometimes clean, and

sometimes disinfect, but rarely do they help any skin disease get better. Their drying effect can greatly aggravate psoriasis, especially that on the extremities.

In general, if a patient with psoriasis has a tendency toward dryness on the arms and legs, I demand that he or she use nothing but gentle, superfatted soaps because of their mildness and moisturizing aspects. I also advise the patient to bathe (or shower) no more than twice a week, maximum. In between, spot-bathing can be done (see Chapter 19).

DERMALERT

If you have psoriasis, frequent washing will only make it worse.

Lotions help, especially if they have cortisone in them, but usually they must be compounded by your dermatologist to get them strong enough to help. Your dermatologist can see your spots, determine what they need, and mix a lotion tailor-made for *your* psoriasis, if necessary. But the moisturizing effect of over-the-counter lotions such as Complex 15 is obvious. They soften the lesions nicely if used frequently enough. If your dryness is tremendously excessive, you might ask your doctor for a prescription for a lotion called Lac-Hydrin. This lotion sometimes causes a little stinging, but it is quite helpful in removing scale and moisturizing the legs and other tough areas.

Heads—Toughest to Treat

Q: I've had thick psoriasis in my scalp for years and was given a treatment lotion, but I was not as faithful in applying it as I should have been. My doctor said he could not refill it without seeing me. What can I use? I've got long white hair and I don't want it discolored.

A: Severe scalp psoriasis is one of the most challenging diseases the skin can develop. It's tough! One of my patients came in with "scale so thick on my scalp that I sometimes can't see the hairs within it." I thought this patient was kidding until I peered through his hair onto a scalp covered with about a half inch of thick, whitish, sheetlike scale which nearly covered his scalp from one side to the other.

"What have you been doing to your scalp?" I asked.

"Well, it itches, Doc," he said, "and when it itches, I scratch it!"

"What do you use to do your scratching," I asked, "a garden rake?"

"You're close, Doc. Actually, and don't laugh when I tell you this," Jim said, "but I use our poodle's metal hairbrush to remove the scales!"

I fell back against the wall grabbing my chest and gasped. "A metal hairbrush! Look Jim," I explained, "nothing could be worse than scratching off those scales with a sharp, stiff metal brush." I told Jim that any irritation of psoriatic skin causes *new* plaques of psoriasis. This "Koebner reaction" often happens in minor scratches and wounds and on knees and elbows where friction is greatest (and, in fact, where *psoriasis* is greatest).

Almost every dermatologist has seen patients like Jim who have been scratching with hat pins, brushes, fingernails, nail files, pencils, and anything else they can get their hands on, not realizing that they're pouring gasoline on the fire of their disease.

I realize full well that itching is a very disagreeable sensation which demands that one scratch. But there's a way to do this which is less harmful and actually applies the medicine at the same time. I've covered it in my kiddie chapter, but I'll mention it again. Put a cortisone lotion or any of the cortisone medications your doctor may have given you on your flat finger pad and rub it into the spot that itches, rather than using a fingernail or other sharp object. This does not damage the skin, and you'll actually treat it repeatedly throughout the day any time it itches. In fact, the itching can be said to be your tiny alarm clock reminding you when to treat your psoriasis! Be sure to *ask your doctor* if this would be appropriate for use with your medication.

Most cortisone medications do not discolor the hair. Occasionally your doctor might choose to use thin cortisone lotions occluded with a plastic shower cap at nighttime to increase their potency. Studies show that this can make your medicine 50 to

100 times more potent, but do not do it unless your doctor specifically instructs you to do so.

Another agent you might try is Baker's P&S lotion. Used every night or every other night, this lotion will very effectively remove scales without your having to pull or scratch them off. Rub about thirty drops into the scalp at nighttime. Baker's P&S is a little tough to wash out in the morning, but it is a very, very effective scale remover.

Most patients have heard about the effective use of tar and tar shampoos on scalp psoriasis. Tar shampoos such as Pentrax, DHS Tar, X-seb-T, Dermalab X5T, Ionil T Plus (which I like best), and many others are very effective treatments for those with brown or black hair, but for anyone with gray, white, or blond hair, they can cause quite a bit of golden-orange tinting. So if you want to try a tar shampoo, and you have white or gray hair, then you should try Iocon shampoo. It does not commonly discolor even these light shades.

Psoriasis shampoos are meant to be scalp *treatments*. So they should be lathered once, rinsed off, lathered again, and left on for five to seven minutes while the medicine in the shampoo has a chance to work. After you have used psoriasis shampoos, you may use a rinse or conditioner of your choice on your scalp, because the treatment from the shampoo has already been accomplished. Keep in mind, too, that a good smoothening rinse is wise to use because it will make it easier to comb your hair. The rinse removes the hair-to-hair friction, and this results in less trauma to the scalp, which could induce more psoriasis. The two most effective rinses are Ionil Rinse and Small Miracle by Clairol.

DERMALERT

Remember the Koebner (pronounced KEB-ner) phenomenon in psoriasis. Any scratch or chronically irritated spot can turn into a new plaque of psoriasis. Since the new lesion of psoriasis is likely to itch, scratching will cause it to get even worse. This starts a vicious psoriasis-causing circle. If you have psoriasis, take *tender loving care* of your skin!

Ear Psoriasis

Q: I have psoriasis on my body, but it's the psoriasis in my *ears* which drives me crazy. The itching is unbearable. One of my closest friends says that I scratch my ears so much that he thinks I was born on my index finger and my right ear. What can I do? Please send me a prescription, quickly!

A: Unfortunately, psoriasis loves ears. But over the years I've found a treatment which is nearly always able to clear ear canal psoriasis: Halog solution. It's applied with a Q-tip to the ear canal as if you were actually painting the walls of the canal itself. The drops are put on the Q-tip (two or three drops will do), never dropped right into the ear. Many of us use this technique, so take this book to a dermatologist and ask whether you can try it. If it works, you've got it made! If not, you've put yourself in touch with a source of help who can advise you on what else you can use. During the acute stages of ear canal psoriasis, the Halog treatment is usually needed twice a day, with the frequency tapering off as you improve. However, take care to heed the old adage, "never put anything in your ear smaller than a football!" *Never* use a wooden-shafted cotton swab, and never put anything far into your ear. To do so is to invite disaster if you slip and damage your eardrum.

The PUVA Promise—Some Good News, Some Bad

Q: I have psoriasis on my hands and feet. I am now taking tetracycline for this, but the problem recurred even while I was taking the medicine. Is there a medication which will prevent the recurrence? What about the new light therapy?

A: Psoriasis of the palms and soles, or palmoplantar psoriasis, is one of the most difficult and painful types of psoriasis. For some reason, a small percentage of patients get these predominantly small pus pockets and scale on the palms and soles rather than the usual body skin-type lesions.

While antibiotics sometimes help, it's often necessary to use cortisone topically for long periods and even internally on a periodic basis to keep this settled down. Of course, we would all like to get away from internal cortisone as much as possible because of its side effects, and recently a development has occurred in psoriasis therapy which has allowed us to do that.

The new treatment is called PUVA. I mentioned it in Chapter 10 in regard to a type of hair loss called alopecia areata. PUVA stands for *p*soralen plus *u*ltraviolet-*A* light therapy. This technique is called *photochemotherapy* because the chemical (psoralen) makes the skin much more photosensitive. The medicine is given two hours before the patient undergoes controlled light exposure in order to give it time to lodge in the skin.

In photochemotherapy, the active drug binds to the DNA of the epidermis. You'll remember that the epidermis is the exact area where psoriasis occurs. This drug attracts ultraviolet light and stops the rapid multiplication of these cells which cause the thick scale and redness of the disease. Special precautions, tests, and light-tight glasses must be used with this treatment, and it's necessary to get two to three treatments a week at the onset. Ask your doctor about this therapy and its possible complications.

DERMALERT

PUVA therapy can clear almost every severe case of psoriasis. But the risks must be considered before you undergo this treatment.

Q: My daughter is being given the PUVA light treatments by an Ohio dermatologist. At the present time she's pregnant with her second child. Will pregnancy have any effect on the psoriasis?

A: Sometimes pregnancy does help psoriasis. However, the course of psoriasis during pregnancy is so variable that an accurate prediction of her course during her pregnancy cannot be made.

More important, however, is the fact that the psoralens she's now taking for the PUVA treatments is listed in the package insert as "Pregnancy Category C." Animal reproduction studies have not been conducted with psoralens. It is also not known whether psoralens can cause fetal harm when administered to a pregnant woman or if psoralens can affect reproduction capacity. In view of this "warning," I don't put any pregnant psoriatics on the drug. I assume that your daughter's dermatologist has weighed the risks, and the two of them have made what they consider to be an appropriate decision for her case.

To avert some of the difficulties with this treatment, some dermatologists are now using psoralens topically. This avoids the various complications of dosing the total body surface with the potent light, when only a fraction of the skin may be involved. There's no sense in exposing the skin to unnecessary damage in areas which do not have psoriasis. It also averts the need to wear protective glasses after the treatments. With systemic photo-chemotherapy, they must be worn during sun exposure for twenty-four hours after UVA treatments. This is because the psoralen binds to the protein in the lens of the eye, and may cause damage (cataracts) if light of the UVA wavelength strikes it. PUVA treatment has been approved by the FDA for use in severe psoriatics.

The Costs of Treatment

Q: I am miserable with psoriasis from head to toe, front to back, and I cannot afford the constant cost to treat this. What can I do for myself? Is there anything less expensive than all the medicines that dermatologists use?

A: Your question occurs to every psoriatic from time to time if they have more than just the minimum of skin disease. Unfortunately, the cost of modern-day medicine is not inexpensive, especially with regard to the cortisone compounds and other strange medicines we use so often in dermatology. However, an intensive psoriasis treatment program does provide the patient the ability to keep working and lead a productive life. In that sense, it can be said to be well worth the expense.

I have suggested on occasion that psoriasis patients go to university clinics or try to obtain public aid for psoriasis, but I have more or less stopped doing this. You see, most public assistance programs will only supply the weakest of medications to patients with skin diseases. This is true in Kentucky, where the most potent medication we can get through regular medical assistance programs is 1% hydrocortisone which, in treating psoriasis, is just about completely ineffective. Occasionally, however, in cases of severe need, exceptions to the rules are made, especially if your doctor will go to the trouble to request special help for you from your state agencies. Ask your doctor; it's certainly worth a try.

So we come full circle right back to the private dermatologist who handles the brunt of psoriasis treatment in this country. Most doctors are reasonable people, and it is often possible to budget payments for dermatologic care and for medications; discuss it with your dermatologist. It is possible that he or she may modify your treatment, follow-up regimen, and medications in order to alleviate your costs somewhat.

There are also some very inexpensive medications which, although potentially hazardous in some ways, do have the benefit of being less expensive. Methotrexate is one of these (see the following section).

Methotrexate—Two-Edged Sword

Q: I would like to know what you think of a medicine for psoriasis called methotrexate. I take eight of them on one day each week. Can they cause internal organ damage?

A: Years ago methotrexate (MTX), a medicine ordinarily used to treat cancer patients, was found to help psoriasis significantly when given by injection or by mouth in nearly every patient who took it.

However, after a while it was noted that some patients on MTX were starting to show changes in their liver, the organ which helps break down drugs and waste products in the body. Those patients who did incur liver damage were usually getting the MTX on a daily basis, whereas those who got the tablets on a once-a-week schedule incurred fewer problems. Now most patients are taking the pills as you do, once a week. Liver damage can still occur, and so can other reactions, such as depression of the blood cell count, so that a close follow-up is mandatory. Usually, the dermatologist will want to have a gastroenterologist or a liver specialist perform a liver biopsy before starting methotrexate. This allows your dermatologist to document whether you have a normal liver prior to the onset of MTX therapy. Periodic, sometimes weekly, lab exams are performed by dermatologists in order to follow closely any changes in liver or blood function. And no alcohol should be ingested during MTX therapy.

But the medicine *does* work. And if you're interested in finding out more about MTX therapy for psoriasis, talk to your dermatologist, who should discuss thoroughly all the possible advantages and disadvantages (complications) of the medicine. It's not an easy drug to use, and patients taking MTX have to be carefully monitored. I urge you to cooperate with your doctor's recommendations in this regard.

Psoriatic Penile Plaques

Q: I have quite severe psoriasis spots on the head of my penis. These spots get much worse after intercourse and take a long time to heal. Sometimes the tiny scales pull off and bleed profusely. Intercourse is really tough sometimes, because I'm so concerned about making my psoriasis worse. Is there any help for this besides abstinence?

A: Discuss this with your dermatologist and relate frankly what is happening. Intercourse is a type of irritation which can induce a Koebner reaction right on the head of the penis (glans). The friction causes minor irritation, which is followed, over the next few days, by new and/or thicker psoriasis plaques.

Your doctor will put you on medications, possibly a special, gentle medication for this soft skin area, which can help alleviate your condition. Adequate lubrication in the vaginal canal is also essential to keeping psoriasis-inducing friction to a minimum. Use plenty of K-Y Jelly, a water washable lubricant, as a friction preventer. Some dermatologists also suggest that a cortisone compound be applied to the head of the penis prior to intercourse so that the lesions may be partially blocked from forming. However, the treatment for genital psoriasis is not perfect, and occasional bouts of abstinence may be necessary to allow healing.

DERMALERT

Good lubrication during intercourse is vital for a psoriatic with genital lesions. This may decrease a tendency to produce new, thick, scaly spots.

Nerves, Cancer, and Psoriasis

Q: You said that the skin was making itself too rapidly in psoriasis spots. Does that mean that it's a type of cancer? Is it cancer of the blood? Do nerves causes psoriasis?

A: Psoriasis has nothing to do with cancer or blood diseases, except that a few of the treatments are somewhat the same for both diseases. But I think there really is something to the fact that some psoriasis patients get better if they are taken out of their stressful day-to-day environment. This was vividly demonstrated to me by a professor of dermatology at the Medical College of Georgia who suggested, "Joe, I'd like you to put Mr. Orvine in the hospital for a few days and do nothing for him, but feed him and give him a place to excrete."

"Don," I said, "you've been working far too hard teaching us residents everything we need to know. I really think you must have lost your mind! Would you like me to run over and grab a shrink for you to talk to?"

"Joe, your touble is that you've got no faith," Don replied. "Trust me for a change, Joe, and see what happens."

"But Don," I exclaimed, "he'll get psoriasis *everywhere* if we just put him in bed and not treat him!"

"Trust me," Don said, "just trust me."

"You're the boss," I said, thinking how strange it was that such a superb clinician should go crazy so suddenly.

So we admitted the 70-year-old man with generalized red psoriasis and tremendous scale everywhere, put him to bed, fed him, and did not apply one stitch of medicine other than to give him anti-itch medicines by mouth.

Amazingly, over the next few days, our elderly patient's scaling decreased, as did his redness, and clear spots of normal-looking skin began peeping through the large areas of psoriasis.

"Don," I admitted, "I'm frankly amazed!"

"I'm not a believer in stress reduction helping *much* in dermatology," Don said, "but in psoriasis, it really has a terrific effect."

"*Touché!*" I exclaimed.

Since then, I've found it to be a constant truth that patients do better when their stress is reduced. This can mean trying to rearrange work so that it's less disagreeable and less stressful, or it can involve other stress reduction techniques, but severe psoriatics should surely try it.

DERMALERT

> Psoriasis is one of the few diseases in which stress has a major effect upon the course of the problem. Any stress-lowering technique effectively used can lessen psoriasis lesions.

Itching

Q: I am 59 years old, and I've had psoriasis since I was in high school. Now I have scales and terrible itching on my right eyelid, a spot on the back of my neck, and even some in my hair. It seems to go away a little bit for a while, and then it comes back, but usually in different places. How can I stop the itching?

A: You've heard me talk about the Koebner reaction, in which more psoriasis is caused by scratching. To prevent this, the important thing, as you've pointed out, is to get rid of the itching. Usually, when the psoriasis starts to improve, the itching does too. This means that you must apply faithfully any medication your dermatologist has given you. Then as your psoriasis gets better, so will your itching.

As a help for the itching in the meantime, I suggest antihistamines such as Atarax and Tavist, which can calm the itching significantly while you are waiting for the spots to heal.

Of course, other treatments besides cortisone can be of help to psoriasis. These include the tar-type medications with or without ultraviolet light. Usually tar is applied overnight, and an ultraviolet treatment is given the next day, but, more recently, modifications of the old tar derivatives have appeared for dermatologists' use.

One of these tar derivatives is a medicine called Drithocreme, an imported anthralin medication from England. Anthralin, while staining and sometimes irritating, can speed the healing of psoriasis tremendously. There are even types of anthralin, called Lasan Pomade and Dritho-Scalp, which can be rubbed into the scalp at nighttime to improve the scalp disease. It's messy and can definitely discolor hair, so you should get exact instructions from your dermatologist before you begin to use this prescription medicine.

The Dead Sea Treatment

Q: I've heard that there is a place in Israel that can cure my psoriasis. How do I get there?

A: The place of which you speak is called the Dead Sea Psoriasis Treatment Center. This clinic is tremendously effective in obliterating psoriasis for extended periods.

The technique used there is quite simple. The place is organized like a European spa and consists basically of a very relaxing atmosphere, sunbathing, and Dead Sea saltwater soaks. Why does it work better than any other psoriasis treatment? Because the Dead Sea has certain minerals in it which are helpful to the healing of psoriasis. Although the reason why salts and minerals help is still being worked out, its beneficial effects indeed seem to hold true for most psoriasis patients.

The most important part in the Dead Sea regimen is the sunshine. Since the Dead Sea is the lowest topographical point on the earth's surface, the sunlight reaching the patients has been filtered through all the various cloud and atmospheric layers, so

that almost all of the nonhelpful rays are gone. In other words
(and more technically), patients here are getting nearly pure UVA
light instead of the combined UVA, UVB, and UVC which most
of us get in daylight sunshine.

Note that the UVA light that these patients get helps heal their
psoriasis without their having to take psoralens by mouth. You'll
remember this in relationship to the PUVA discussion we had
earlier.

So is it worth it for you to travel to the Dead Sea Psoriasis
Treatment Center? Probably not. The treatment is very expensive,
takes several weeks of your time, and your remission is usually
only for six to eight months. It does work, but it's not a cure.

If you would like to obtain more information, you should write:

Dr. Willy Avrach
P. O. Box 20
Savyon, Israel

Infantile Psoriasis

Q: At six months of age, our grandson started with a case of
psoriasis, and it recurs often. Is this unusual?

A: Unfortunately, it's not unusual enough. I've seen my
youngest case of psoriasis at six *weeks*! The age of onset seems
not to be at all predictable. But it surely is a lot tougher to treat
in babies, because their tender skins won't tolerate some of the
more potent medicines which work so well in adults.

Psoriasis in History

Q: Weren't there some strange things used in the past for
treating psoriasis?

A: Until a few years ago, low-dose arsenic had been used
successfully in treating difficult psoriasis. But since arsenic causes
internal cancers and other problems many years after its administration, its practical use was restricted to the elderly, who would

not be expected to encounter these late appearing sequelae during their lifetimes. This just demonstrates how psoriasis therapy differs, depending on the age groups under consideration.

You should now understand a lot more about psoriasis and its treatment. The general public understands so little about the disease that prejudice and preconceived notions run rampant, making the psoriatic's life miserable. If I've dulled those prejudices even a little, I'll consider this book a success.

17

Fry Now, Pay Later*— Sun Cancers, Melanomas, and Moles

Over 600,000 cases of skin cancer happen in this country *every year*, making it the most common of all types of cancer. Over 17,000 cases of malignant melanoma (the most deadly form of skin cancer) are discovered each year, resulting in over 5,000 deaths. And why is this problem so massive in proportions? *Sunlight!* It's nearly the sole cause of two major types of skin cancers, and the probable cause in many of the melanoma cases.

But people still love to lie in the sun.

DERMALERT

Sunlight causes more cancer than any other known carcinogen.

As a child, I was guilty of my own sun indiscretions. I remember a radio contest one year in which we all taped our backs with the call letters of an Akron station. The winner (not me) was the guy

* Used with permission of the American Cancer Society.

who got the greatest contrast between his sizzled back and the baby-white skin below the letters. Nowadays, we dermatologists must contend with much more than a single dark tan. We now have that "wonderful" invention, the tanning salon, to keep the damage coming year round.

Tanning Salons

Q: How safe are tanning salons? Can they actually be harmful to your skin? Are they worse than the sun?

A: Frankly, going to a tanning salon is an open and frontal assault on your skin. The American Academy of Dermatology, in 1979, issued a general alert concerning the practice. Tanning salon patrons may, through the years, develop many more skin cancers because of this intense, direct exposure to the exact wavelengths of light that a person *shouldn't* have.

Worse than the sun? Certainly! These booths emit the dangerous, cancer-causing rays at a very close distance, giving a much more concentrated exposure than ordinary sunlight.

Tanning Beds

Q: But what about the "new" booths, the so-called European system? They're much safer, aren't they?

A: In response to all the advertisements touting these "tanning beds" as safer, the American Academy of Dermatology's Task Force on Photobiology has recently issued a release giving their views on the new booths. They can actually cause a host of serious problems, including cataracts, skin cancer, accelerated aging, potentiation of the cancer-causing effects of regular sunlight, and, believe it or not, possibly even changes in the body's *immune system*!

A patient of mine gave his opinion on those dangers, when, after I explained the complications of tanning beds, he exclaimed, "Wow, you mean they can really cause all that? No wonder they look so much like coffins!"

Stay away from them! Your poor skin has enough to contend with, just with all the sunlight chemicals and natural pollutants, let alone this source of *artificial* pollutant, which can, in fact, be 1,000 times more damaging than regular sunlight!

Q: But don't we need a certain amount of natural sunlight on our skin in order to process vitamin D, and for other health reasons?

A: You'll get plenty of vitamin D from milk supplementation and other dietary sources without needing sunlight to process it for you. And the sun is definitely *not* needed for other health reasons. The little bit we all get walking to and from the car is a hundred times more than we need.

Q: But I always *look* so healthy when I'm tanned!

A: Beauty, in this regard, is definitely in the eye of the beholder. I think you look quite damaged, myself. Tanning is the first and best indicator that sun damage *has already been done* to your skin. While the tan protects you somewhat on future exposure to the sun, it can't stop the real damage from building up cumulatively—year after year, after wrinkled, cancerous year!

DERMALERT

Tanning is the quintessential indicator of sun damage.
When you're tanned, you're damaged.

Sunlight and the Skin

In the old days of bonnets and parasols, women would have cursed every minute they were forced to be in the sun. They seem to have known what it would do to them. But somewhere along the line, women, and men too, forgot about the horrendous things sunlight does to skin. Lately, I've been encouraging everyone to join what I call my "Tan is Tacky Club," to try to reeducate people about sun damage.

I once watched a movie being filmed in the Arizona desert, and I was amazed at the lengths to which the young, smooth-skinned actresses would go in order *not* to be in the sunlight. There was a whole crew of men with umbrellas assigned to shield them from the bright sun. After all, those actresses knew that their very careers depended on the avoidance of sun wrinkles. Oh, if we would all realize that fact!

Q: I've heard a lot over the last few years about the ozone layer slowly being destroyed by high-flying jets and by aerosol sprays. Who cares?

A: Ozone is the only substance which keeps us from sizzling in the sunlight like so many potato chips! It's the wonderful stuff made by lightning that absorbs most of the damaging ultraviolet rays of the sun. Fluorinated hydrocarbon sprays break down the ozone, letting the sun shine in. That's why everyone was anxious to stop them from being used several years ago. Now, almost all the sprays are pressurized with other gases such as isobutane, which are harmless to the ozone layer.

Unhappily, aerosol sprays are not the only sources of damage to the ozone layer. We've still got a problem with high-flying commercial and military jets which could result in more skin cancers in the future. Later in this chapter, we'll discuss how to protect yourself even with less ozone.

DERMALERT

As the ozone layer of our atmosphere decreases, skin cancers will increase radically in upcoming years. That makes the use of various types of sunscreen hyper-critical.

Let's talk some more about general and specific points regarding sunlight.

Q: If you spend a lot of time in the sun when you are young, do you show signs of aging earlier in life?

A: You bet! Sunlight is the prime cause of the aged look as the years pass. I often use this fact in order to convince patients to protect their skin from sun. It seems as if very few people listen if I say, "You're going to get skin cancer if you don't change your sunbathing habits." But if I tell them, "Sunbathing will make you look like a wrinkled old prune," they'll listen to me almost every time.

So to accomplish my purpose of shading as much skin as possible, I'll appeal to vanity any time. If it works, use it!

Know how to prove to yourself that sunlight causes the aged look? Take a look at the neck skin of a farmer or a sailor, and then look at the covered chest skin of the same person. The neck skin is wrinkled and coarse, just like football leather, but the covered skin is as smooth as a newborn baby's bottom. And yet that skin's the exact same age as the wrinkled skin.

Q: Wouldn't I get the same wrinkles anyway, sooner or later?

A: Of course not! There's no reason to count on wrinkles, any more than you'd count on any other personal tragedy (which is what we skin doctors think wrinkles are). If you avoid alcohol, is it likely that you'll still get cirrhosis? If you don't eat like a whale, is it likely you'll get fat? Of course not, and the same holds true for sun damage.

Of course, there are some gravity-type wrinkles which still occur, but they're really minor compared with the intense wrinkling of sun damage.

Q: Can lying out in the sun really be the cause of skin cancer? How about genetics? Don't some families have it, some not?

A: Again, the distribution of the problem ought to tell you what causes it. The vast majority of skin cancers occur on sun-exposed skin. If you could spend just one day with me in my office, you'd be convinced of this simple fact forever. If you could just see how many faces and noses we have to whittle on to remove skin cancers, you would never doubt it. As I carved off the tip of the nose of an *18-year-old* with skin cancer one day, she whispered, "I'll not fail to listen to *you* again!"

It's definitely true that some families tend to get what I prefer to call "sun cancer" a lot more easily and earlier than other families. These are the Scotch-Irish, Nordic, and Scandinavian peoples with blue eyes, fair skin, and red hair. They are at tremendously greater risk than darker-skinned people, but still, dark-skinned Mediterranean types certainly can get skin cancers, and often do. It's just that they are afforded a little more natural protection in the form of melanin skin pigmentation.

DERMALERT

The most susceptible people to sun cancer are fair-skinned, blue-eyed, red-haired, blonde, Scotch-Irish, Celtic, Nordic, and Scandinavian peoples. For these people, a little bit of sun can be deadly.

Q: If a woman of 55 years of age has been sunbathing all her life, can she still sunbathe without damaging her skin?

A: That damage she's been incurring all these years has never left her. It's cumulative, that is, it builds up over a person's entire lifetime, just like x-ray therapy. Every sun-exposed skin cell carries the genetic damage of each and every exposure. I wish it did go away. Then the number of skin cancers would actually get less with old age, assuming we could finally convince the public to refrain from sunbathing.

But take hope! The cellular sun damage won't fade with time, but your wrinkles might! Researchers have discovered that the sun damage to the dermis, which is responsible for all the fine wrinkles of old age, does indeed lessen with age, if the skin is no longer exposed. To prove this, they've done some rather bizarre tests. They've applied sunscreens to *one-half* of the body of elderly nursing home patients, and rolled them out into the sun day after day. With enough time, biopsy specimens from the skin of the sunscreened side did show *reversal* of the changes leading to wrinkling. It certainly pays to avoid the sun!

DERMALERT

Sun damage builds up throughout one's lifetime. But it may be possible, by avoiding the sun for a period of years, to actually reverse the damage induced by the sun's rays.

Q: When's the best time to lie out in the sun?

A: About 11:30 at night. Really there's no good time to destroy your skin. We do know that the worst times are from 10 a.m. to 2 p.m. And, of course, the sun's much hotter in southern climes, because, due to the earth's curvature, you're lying physically closer to the sun. In tropical areas one can get "cutaneously cooked" and "dermally done" in just a matter of minutes.

Q: You sure gripe a lot about the sun, but there's one place I *can't* avoid it. When I am in my car the sun is extremely intense through the windows. It hits me regardless of where I sit. Any way to avoid this?

A: I've got great news for you. Sunlight through window glass is completely harmless! The damaging part, called UVB, is filtered out as the light strikes the glass. Its energy is transformed into great amounts of radiant heat which streams into the car. That's why the interior temperature of a car can reach 120 to 130°F quite easily, on just a moderately warm day. It can become a veritable solar *furnace* in there. (No wonder so many animals die when left in cars!)

Now think of this. That terrific energy would have been available to damage and irrevocably alter the genetic material of your skin cells had you been directly exposed. That's even one more fact which should convince you to stay out of the sun's direct rays.

Q: I was working in my kitchen with the TV on when I heard you speak on skin cancer. I thought I had nothing to worry about until you mentioned "itch." I never thought a skin cancer would itch. Well, I nearly broke a bone getting to a paper and pen to take down information on where to write you. I've *got* an itchy place! Please tell me why a skin cancer would itch.

A: Itching has been discovered to be one of the cardinal signs of skin cancer.

Have your dermatologist check your skin spot if it:

1. Itches
2. Changes in color
3. Bleeds
4. Won't heal
5. Forms a scar for which there was no injury
6. Turns red, white, blue, or black
7. Develops a surrounding halo of whiteness

8.   Has uneven pigment or notches in the pigment's edges

9.   Ulcerates or erodes

You should examine your entire skin surface once yearly for any spots which display any of these signs. If you've got any of these signs of skin cancer, *run*, don't walk, to your dermatologist for a checkup.

Itching in skin cancers has always been somewhat of a mystery. We're just now starting to figure out why it happens. Itching is one of the few ways that skin has of calling attention to itself when something is wrong. In fact, itching may be caused by the body's immune system. If the immune system detects changes in cells which make those cells look foreign, as cancer cells would, for instance, it calls out various destroyer cells to try to eliminate the invaders. It often does this successfully, too. There are noted cases of virtual resolution of cancers, including skin cancers, which look like "miracle cures" because of the effective surveillance of the immune system. Researchers think, in fact, that each person develops many cancers over a lifetime, and that the immune system wipes them out very effectively.

DERMALERT

Itching is one of the most significant signs of incipient skin cancer. If you have a spot that itches, your skin is trying to tell you that something is changing.

So itching should be a cardinal signal that something has gone wrong in the skin. Heed the signal. You may only get one chance.

Q: How does a physician know that a spot is okay by just looking at and examining it?

A: Your question reminds me of the fifties' joke about the violinist who stops a Beatnik on a New York street corner and asks, "Hey, buddy, how do I get to Carnegie Hall?"

"Practice, man, *practice!*" the Beatnik answers.

It takes a *lot* of learning and practice to make the judgment calls on tens and tens of lesions every day. I guess that's why it takes so long to become a dermatologist.

Sunspots

Q: I have a small place on my cheek about the size of my little fingernail. It gets rough and scales off, and then it will be smooth for a while, and then go through the same thing. It isn't really sore unless I pick the skin off. I know I shouldn't do this, but it's tough to resist. I'm 73 years old. What is it?

A: The problem you're describing may be an actinic keratosis (AK). This is usually a reddish, slightly scaly spot on a light-exposed area of the skin, such as yours. They begin somewhat brown in color, progress to red, and then get slightly to moderately scaly. The importance of actinic keratoses is that they can turn into skin cancers, and often do. Experts feel as many as 10 percent of AKs will, sooner or later, turn into skin cancers, usually of the squamous cell type (more about this later).

DERMALERT

Ordinary skin does not get red and scaly. Redness or scaliness in isolated patches is a prime symptom of a premalignant sunspot called *actinic keratosis*.

Actinic keratoses do scale off from time to time, and in fact, that's what may keep people from getting them treated earlier. They think that since their spot peeled off once or twice before, it'll keep peeling off in layers until it's all gone. Usually, this is untrue, because no matter how many times the spot peels off, the underlying cells which make the scaly part remain to remake the scale.

However, as much as I hate to say it, picking them off doesn't really make them any worse. More than one dermatologist feels that shaving is responsible for the very few AKs we see on the cheeks of men, while the foreheads, bald spots, ears, neck, and hands are often covered with them. I'm *not* advising you to try to pick off your premalignant lesions, however. Get them checked!

In my office, AKs are usually removed by cryosurgery—spraying on liquid nitrogen to freeze them and make them peel off. The process stings a little, but usually leaves no sign that the AK was ever there. Cryosurgery is extremely useful for a limited number of lesions, and usually eliminates them permanently in the areas sprayed.

However, if we take the example of actinic keratoses on the face, the entire face was exposed for years to about the same amount of light, so that in areas which were not frozen, we could expect new lesions to arise with time. This is called the "field theory" in dermatology, indicating that the lesions can arise anywhere in the field which has received the damage (in this case, from the sun).

Q: I have a large brown "mole" which my doctor called senile keratosis. Is that the same as an AK? My bra rubs this lesion and I am concerned about that causing malignancy. Does it?

A: AK is not really the same as a senile keratosis. A senile keratosis is a seborrheic keratosis (see Chapter 20). They are not premalignant.

Constant rubbing of a spot used to be thought to cause cancer. It does not. What it does cause is irritation, which can result in a lot of confusion and anxiety when the spot is seen by a physician. If you'll remember, redness, scaling, bleeding, and so on are all signs of skin cancer, and that's also how doctors tell if a spot's malignant or not. Therefore, if a place is irritated by clothing constantly, a physician might look at the spot and think it's a skin cancer, when, in fact, it's not. This may prompt the doctor to take off a much larger piece of skin than necessary as a precaution, in case it's proved to be a skin cancer. Understand? I hope so. Anyway, the bottom line is that the spot should probably be removed so that it doesn't confuse the picture if it ever does get irritated.

Efudex—The "TMB Cream"

Q: One time you mentioned "TMB cream." What is this used for?

A: As you'll read in Chapter 20, TMBs are marks that result from *too many birthdays*. Certainly this applies, in a way, to AKs. The cream I talked about on the show was Efudex. This potent anticancer drug, called 5-fluorouracil, was discovered quite by accident to have destructive effects on premalignant lesions of the skin, namely, actinic keratoses. When the drug was injected into cancer patients, a curious reddening of their sunspots was noticed, and some of the spots actually faded away permanently. Startled, the researchers tried the drug in a topically applied form which also worked spectacularly on AKs. This drug is now marketed under the brand name Efudex.

The substance will not treat all TMBs, however, and it's a pretty tough treatment program to go through. You see, Efudex works not only on the scaly lesions you can see, but also on the microscopic ones you don't even know are there yet. So patients on Efudex therapy start to get red in all sorts of places they never even suspected they had sunspots before. And the redness, while tolerable, does often get quite severe. The treatment has to be continued for three to six weeks in order to knock out all the premalignant lesions. It's tough to find patients willing to go through the redness and scabbing of this course of therapy, because almost everyone turns out to have three family reunions, an audience with the pope, and an appearance on *Good Morning America* scheduled during the proposed treatment period! If the treatment is stopped too early, only a fraction of the lesions will be wiped out.

Sunlight makes the Efudex reaction much more severe, so most patients are cautioned to perform this treatment only in the wintertime, when their sun exposure could be expected to be at a minimum. That makes it even tougher for those who would like to leave town on vacation while their faces are red from the medicine—they can't go to a sunny area.

Q: I've used that sunspot cream before, but after all the spots lit up with the chemical, my normal skin, even in clothing-covered areas, got all red and blistery! What happened?

A: As with all medicines, an allergy can develop to Efudex. When this happens, the reaction you describe is seen in the normally shaded areas. This is a true contact allergy, and will probably prohibit the use of Efudex in your case. Your dermatologist can tell you how to do a patch test or a use test in order to see if you're allergic or not.

Basal Cell Carcinoma—
The Most Common Cancer

Q: I'm a frequent sunbather, and I've developed a spot on my shoulder which has a whitish bump and blisters on it. Inside the spot there are some blackish flecks, like moles. Is there any need for concern? What could this be?

A: There's a good chance that you have the most common of all skin cancers, a basal cell carcinoma (BCC). There are 600,000 of these spots which occur in this country every *year*, making it by far the most common form of cancer.

BCCs are slow-growing, indolent tumors which, again, don't usually spread to internal organs. They begin as small, flesh-colored, whitish, or even slightly red bumps on the skin. They very often are discrete, isolated bumps, but occasionally take on a diffuse appearance that's much more difficult to eradicate. This particular form is called the *morphea*, or diffuse-type, BCC. The bumplike BCCs are called *nodular basal cells*. Often they will ulcerate and bleed, forming recurrent crusts. This is the classic sign the American Cancer Society tells us about in their warning, "Beware of a sore that doesn't heal!"

Bleeding is usual for BCCs because of the many tiny blood vessels which develop over the surface of these tumors. They can be seen quite easily on close inspection of a BCC with a hand magnifying lens.

Some BCCs look like depressed areas in the skin, often surrounded by a tiny raised border. Occasional ones even have a "chewed-out" appearance that the very descriptive early dermatologists called "rodent ulcers," after their resemblance to the ragged, punched-out border of a rat bite.

DERMALERT

Bumps on the skin with tiny blood vessels running over them are very often basal cell carcinoma.

Almost universally caused by sunlight, BCCs are dangerous because they expand locally, and invade, by direct extension, adjacent structures. This becomes a matter of serious concern when these lesions are located next to important structures such as the nose, eyes, and ears.

BCCs are removed in much the same ways as SCCAs (squamous cell carcinoma). In the elderly, and in persons who would not be expected to tolerate surgery very well, radiation therapy can be used very adequately.

Q: I had a basal cell carcinoma eleven years ago which was surgically removed, and it has recurred. Is there a way to have it removed so it won't recur again?

A: There sure is! The most effective method for removal of a recurrent skin cancer is a relatively new surgical technique, Mohs' microscopically controlled excision. Mohs' surgery involves the exact mapping of the tumor. The lesion is cut off in horizontal sections, each of which is labeled and sent individually to the dermatopathologist for examination. If any of the sections still have skin cancer in them, then just a little more adjacent skin in *that area* is cut out again. This is repeated until all the sections submitted are tumor-free.

Mohs' surgery results in the highest possible cure rate for BCCs and SCCAs. But it's not necessary for simple first-time-treated tumors, and it's considerably more complicated and more expensive than conventional surgery. Also, it's not available everywhere, so your dermatologist will discuss its need and availability in your case.

Squamous Cell Skin Cancer

Q: I am deviled and bedeviled with squamous-type skin cancers, three of which I have had over a period of years and have had removed surgically. Is there an ointment or salve to clear up this kind of skin cancer?

A: Squamous cell carcinoma (SCCA) is the second most common type of skin cancer dermatologists treat. It's caused by continuous sun damage to the mid- and upper epidermis, or topmost skin layer. These lesions are important because they are the ones which result directly from AKs. They grow by local extension, and usually do not spread through the lymphatic drainage system, or the blood vessel network. In other words, for most types of SCCAs, local surgical removal will take care of them.

Squamous cancers look like thickened AKs. That is, they frequently have the redness and scaliness of actinic keratoses, but they look more aggressive, with more redness, more scale, and occasionally crusting and bleeding. Usually, they are thick enough to have a harder, or indurated, feel. Squamous cancers usually are not accompanied by the blackish pigment we often see in melanomas, but they can be various shades of brown or brown-red.

Interestingly, the first draft of this part of this book did not contain the above description. I omitted it because I felt that words could not adequately describe what it takes us dermatologists three years to spot and identify accurately. I still believe, even after adding the above information, that you should not try to diagnose your own skin cancers. These morphological signs of skin cancer are added so that you will have any suspicious spot *checked* without delay. So use the signs I list in *Skin Secrets*, but use them as a guide to alert you to see your dermatologist. He or she has the experiential equipment to diagnose your problem.

While the treatment for SCCA is surgical removal, this can include several types of surgery. The first and probably most common type is standard knife removal, in which the spot is cut out, and the edges of the remaining wound are stitched shut. This very effective method results in a linear, or linelike, scar.

DERMALERT

> Squamous cell and basal cell skin cancers usually do not spread to other parts of the body, but they do grow by local extension into vital structures; so they should be taken off as soon as possible.

The second method is by what we call the shave, curettage, and electrodesiccation (C&ED) method. In this technique, the lesion is numbed with a local anesthetic and shaved off tangential to the skin, and the site of the cancer is scraped vigorously with a curved knife blade called a *curette*. (The shaved-off part of the tumor is sent off to the pathologist to confirm its type.) The curette scrapes away any remaining tumor. This scraping procedure is performed on each of three different surgical planes, or levels, and after each of the scrapings, the site of the cancer is thoroughly buzzed with an electric needle to assure that a few more cell layers are killed off each time. This gives a higher cure rate for the procedure. In fact, the 90 to 94 percent cure rate of this so-called C&ED procedure is equal to that of the knife removal technique. This is the type of procedure President Reagan had done on his nose in 1985 for a basal cell cancer. We'll talk about that type shortly.

The third method for removing this type of skin cancer is cryosurgery. A superstrong freeze is delivered to the tumor which kills off the cancer cells. As you might guess, this type of freeze is much deeper than that used to, say, freeze a wart or a seborrheic keratosis as mentioned in Chapter 4. Often, a thermocouple (an implanted thermometer in a needle) is used to monitor the depth of freeze to assure the best treatment of the cancer. It's a detailed procedure, and it results in a fairly severe blister which weeps for a few days, crusts over, and then falls off in four to six weeks.

The scars left from the second and third methods are disk-shaped, and usually somewhat whiter than the surrounding skin. But the methods do provide a good cure rate with as little defect as possible. Many of us use the cryosurgical and C&ED methods for most of the skin cancers we see in the office.

Q: I am 83 years old, and I've had a growth on my lip which has been burned off twice, but nothing seems to help. I used to walk to lunch every day at noon for thirteen years, and maybe that's where I got it. I never knew enough to wear a hat or carry an umbrella, as I do now. What should I do?

A: If you should happen to have an SCCA on your lip, that's a different story. This particular type of squamous cancer *does* occasionally spread to other areas of the body, so it's absolutely critical to get it removed as soon as possible. There is, however another condition, called *actinic cheilitis* (pronounced kigh-LIGHT-is), which is chronic inflammation of the lip due to sun damage. It's the lip equivalent of an actinic keratosis (AK).

DERMALERT

Scaliness on the lower lip is a prime example of a skin cancer waiting to happen. Shield your lips with Eclipse Lip Protectant or Chap Stick 15 SPF lip balm so that the damage does not occur.

Actinic cheilitis may be treated, after biopsy confirmation that no cancer is yet present, by cryosurgery or by Efudex applications. Either one will temporarily cause a sore lip, but it's worth it to get a potentially fatal condition resolved.

For a comparison of basal and squamous skin cancers, see the following table.

CHARACTERISTICS OF BASAL AND SQUAMOUS SKIN CANCERS

	BASAL	SQUAMOUS
Nodule (raised bump)	Frequent	Occasional
Tiny blood vessels on surface	Frequent	Rare
Scaling	Less common	Frequent
Color	Pale, pearly, rarely pigmented	Red or red-brown
Internal spread	Extremely rare	Very rare
Sun-caused	Yes	Yes
Treatment	Varies, multiple	Varies, multiple
Prognosis	Excellent	Excellent
Growth pattern	Slow	Slow
Invades local structures	Yes	Yes
Preceded by actinic keratosis (AK)	No	Yes, usually
Seen in old burn scars	Rarely	Yes, occasionally
Location	Light-exposed areas	Light-exposed areas
"Rodent ulcer"	Often	Rarely
Bleeding	Yes	Less frequently

Q: My dermatologist wants me to get a "lip shave." What's this, and what would I look like? Does it mean that I've hair on my lip?

A: Not at all! You've got a case of fairly severe actinic cheilitis, and your doctor wants to make sure that all those bad cells get taken care of. He or she has asked you to have all the skin on your lower lip removed, or "shaved," so that all the damaged skin is gone. After the shaving off of all the damaged tissue, the soft, moist mucous membrane inside the lip is pulled outward, or "advanced," to form a new, normal-looking lip line. This procedure's marvelous. It relieves you of all your scaliness and premalignant lip spots all at once.

The lip usually heals up beautifully with almost no sign of any previous damage. But remember that the same damage can recur if you again get a lot of sunlight exposure. And the second time around, it's not as easy to find good tissue for the lip shave procedure.

Melanoma

While all skin cancers are important, not all are immediately life-threatening. For instance, the basal cell carcinoma and squamous cell carcinomas we've discussed often take months to years even to become noticeable, and many more years to become life-threatening (the exception to this, obviously, is the tumor which is located near a vital structure, such as a tear duct, ear canal, or eyelid).

But melanoma is a different story. This tumor of pigment cells is life-threatening, by definition, *if it exists*. Except for certain rare instances of regression of melanoma, all melanomas, if left untreated, have the potential to cause the demise of the patient.

Melanoma starts as a collection of just a few pigment cells which multiply in a disorganized fashion. When they are first noticeable, the tiny spot they form is quite thin. It thickens as it grows, pressing deeper and deeper into the dermis below and actually growing into it.

The flat spot thickens progressively into a small lump (nodule).

The thicker the lesion (pathologists actually measure every malignant melanoma, or MM, with a microscopic ruler), the worse the outlook for cure. All MMs have the potential of spreading in three ways: They may grow directly into surrounding structures (direct invasion); they may spread via the lymph system (lymphatic spread); or they may spread through the bloodstream (hematogenous spread). All forms of spread are called *metastases*. Metastases of MM may occur at any time, but are much less likely if the tumor is removed when it's still thin.

"Melanoma" is a word which is derived from the word "melanin." That's the pigmentary material that is responsible for all the various shadings of color in human skin. The melanin is made by special cells called *melanocytes*, which are hidden deep in the base of the uppermost skin layer, the epidermis. While melanocytes ordinarily go about their normal factorylike production of melanin, they can occasionally start to multiply in a greatly disorganized fashion. The tumor that results is the MM.

The crucial fact to remember in melanomas, however, is that timing is ultracritical. If you have any of the symptoms of skin cancers we've discussed, *please* make the investment in this book count and get your dermatologist to check out the suspicious spots.

Q: I recently noticed a sore spot on my back as if I had bumped it. The next morning I noticed it was still hurting. The spot looked to my husband like a blister. We used a bandage until we could get to my doctor, because we didn't have a dermatologist. My doctor didn't want to do anything since it looked infected, and told me to come back in a week so he could see how it was clearing.

After a week, a scab had formed, and there was a light brown, raised mole below. My doctor informed me that it didn't look cancerous, and if it bothered me again, to come back and he'd remove it. Since you're a dermatologist, I was wondering, have you ever had a case like mine?

A: Go see a dermatologist immediately. You may have a malignant melanoma. If you catch it early, it can be readily cured. If you wait, however, you could be in very bad trouble.

DERMALERT

Most melanomas, especially the thin ones, are curable. It's only when a patient waits too long in getting a melanoma checked that a problem results.

Q: What causes melanoma?

A: That's still one of the great mysteries. Apparently there's some disordering of the skin cells' normal multiplication, but what turns on this disorder, or, rather, what cancels out the ordinarily magnificent orderliness with which these cells multiply, is unknown.

However, we're now getting some hints. Melanomas show a surprisingly high occurrence rate on sun-exposed skin, a disturbing fact that is just now becoming apparent. Heretofore, we thought all we really had to worry about because of sun exposure were wrinkles, basal cell carcinomas, and squamous cell carcinomas.

But as the ozone layer decreases further and further, and as the quest for the "great American tan" continues, the incidence of MM has reached over 17,000 *new* cases each year, with about 5,000 deaths yearly from the disease. So we're getting quite a bit more vocal about the deleterious effects of sunshine.

Q: My son has a mole on his hand which is very dark, and it seems to have lighter-colored skin over it. However, deep down under the skin is a black bump. It's been there many years. Should he have this taken off?

A: While it's very possible that the dark spot could be an MM, it's more probably a benign lesion called a *blue nevus*. That's a noncancerous blue-black nodule deep under the skin, the look of which is generally calmer than that of an MM. Also, they don't grow, scab over, crust, bleed, change color, or itch, as BCCs, SCCAs, and MMs do. But because of the pigment, which is apparently deep down in the skin, I would probably biopsy the spot. But it should be checked regardless, so get your son to a dermatologist.

If the lesion does indeed turn out to be a benign blue nevus, at least he'll have it off, and not have to worry about it anymore.

Q: What's a black melanoma? What other kinds are there?

A: Melanomas come in many different colors. They may be

tan, brownish, brown-black, blue-black, black, or even completely colorless without any pigment at all. As they grow, they may have a deep blue shade, indicating pigment deep down in the dermis, or they may be reddish, indicating inflammation (the body's reaction against the tumor), or even white in some areas, indicating regression and resolution of a part of the growth.

The histological type, depth, and thickness are far more important than the color of the tumor. We'll discuss more about thickness and prognosis later.

Q: My husband died of a black melanoma some time ago, and had had quite a few skin cancers removed before the melanoma developed. Is my daughter, who is a sun worshiper, more apt to get melanoma because my husband died of it?

A: Melanomas are somewhat more common in fair-skinned, blue-eyed, red- and blond-haired, Scotch-Irish, English, and Nordic individuals because of their increased sensitivity to damaging sunlight. Your daughter should definitely take that into consideration the next time she goes out to roast herself.

More important, though, is your question about a possible genetic tendency toward MM. There have been some important findings about a special hereditary form of MM. Since 1952, sporadic cases of a condition called *dysplastic nevus syndrome* (DNS) have been found. This is apparently a dominant hereditary characteristic, afflicting several members in a family with strange-looking moles and cutting across generations. As a result of this condition, these individuals have a tremendously high probability of getting MM. That's good enough reason why every person on this planet should have at least one "mole check," as we call it in our office, most urgently in his or her childhood. If it is discovered that a person has DNS, very close follow-up by the dermatologist is recommended, possibly as often as every six months or so.

DERMALERT

You and every immediate relative of a patient with melanoma should be checked for strange moles on the body. Anything suspicious should be biopsied.

The Skin Cancer Foundation now advises that a dermatologist screen every immediate blood relative of melanoma patients in order to spot these DNS lesions more rapidly, and take action at a time when it can really help.

Q: I recently had an MM removed from my arm. I'm in my thirties, and I wondered if you could tell me about the survival statistics on MM.

A: That depends largely on the type, depth, and height of your particular MM. There are several different types, all of which have a different prognosis (expected survival time). The most common type we're seeing these days is the very thin MM, which carries with it the best of all possible prognoses.

For instance, very thin MMs (those with a thickness of less than 0.76 millimeter) have virtually a 100 percent survival rate. However, the prognosis for thick lesions which have penetrated the fat below the skin is dismal. This is the reason why finding MMs early is so very important.

You should discuss your prognosis with your cancer surgeon and dermatologist. They'll be much better able to tell you the details on whether you can expect to be completely rid of the disease.

I've done a lot of preaching concerning the harmful effects of the sun, but as yet I haven't told you too much about how to avoid them. Let's discuss protection in detail.

Sunscreens—The Modern Way to Protect

Q: What's the best sunscreen for fair-skinned people?

A: Sunscreens come in two major types. We're all familiar with the old parasol-and-bonnet concept. That's all our ancestors had to prevent themselves from wrinkling up like prunes in the hot sun. This type of sunscreen is the physical type. It includes long sleeves, and white, reflective clothing to shield the tender skin below.

More recently, a new concept in sun protection has evolved with "parasols in a bottle," or chemical sunscreens. These agents are some of the most remarkable chemicals in human history. They are composed of molecules with a special affinity for sunlight. The thin, protective layer they put down can shield you from 99 percent of the sun's harmful rays, depending on the composition of the chemical sunscreen.

What's the best one? PreSun 15 is the industry standard of excellence. It contains PABA, or para-aminobenzoic acid, the most active sunscreen ever found. Of course there are others with PABA, but, in my opinion, this is the best. You know how to find the best of anything medical? Ask your doctor which one he or she uses. PreSun 15's the one *I* use! Another good one is Sundown 15, especially for swimmers. Others that are supposedly equally as protective include, but are not limited to, Total Eclipse 15, Coppertone Supershade 15, Charles of the Ritz's Bain de Soleil, and Clinique's 15-rated sunscreen.

Q: What're the numbers for?

A: The numbers (called *sun protection factors*, or SPFs) which follow the name of the preparation indicate how much they shield you from the sun. For instance, with no sunscreen at all, the human skin rates a 1. That is, the skin burns in a set number of minutes (the first time) for each person. Now, if that same person, who burns, say in ten minutes on the year's first exposure, wears a number "8" sunscreening lotion, then he or she would have to stay out for 80 (10 X 8) minutes to get the same degree of burn. In other words, the higher the SPF number (up to the federally permitted maximum of 15), the higher the degree of protection.

Q: Which number should I use?

A: The sunscreen manufacturers tell us that each person has to make up his or her own mind regarding the extent of protection needed. We are left to shift for ourselves in determining the amount of damage we want to risk!

I personally believe that all people should give themselves the best possible shot at making it through life "skin cancerless." So use a 15-rated sunscreen every time you'll get significant sun exposure. You might as well take good care of that skin of yours. It may be the only one you'll ever get!

Swimmers, Listen Up!

Q: I lifeguard every summer, and I really need something super to guard my nose. Toward the end of the day at our public pool, my nose looks like a hotdog left one hour in a microwave oven! What do you suggest? Got anything for us swimmers that'll stick on in the water?

A: There's a terrific skin-colored, complete blockout cream, called R.V.Paque, made by the Elder Company. Your pharmacist can order this for you. It's likely that you'll get as much protection as offered by the zinc oxide ointment you lifeguards are so fond of using.

Waterproof sunscreens are quite difficult to come by, but there's a way to make your regular 15-rated sunscreen stay on better in the water. First, apply the liquid about an hour before you'd expect to be in the water, and again about a half hour before exposure. That'll give your sunscreen a chance to soak right into the dead layer of the skin, called the *stratum corneum*. That's the important layer that shields us from the various hazards of our environment.

DERMALERT

Applying your 15-rated sunscreen twice at half-hour intervals before swimming can keep it on much better. Also, daily applications allow a constant layer of it to be present in your skin all the time.

Several years ago, the Johnson & Johnson company developed a sunscreen called Sundown 15, and it contains a film which adheres to the skin, even with water immersion. So it's best for swimmers. Recently it's been tested after four 20-minute swims and found to still hold its 15 SPF rating! Recently PreSun 15 *Creamy* lotion has been found to be virtually waterproof, too. You can buy both sunscreens at the drugstore without a prescription.

Last, and possibly most important, are your poor lips. Nothing takes the beating of lifeguard lips! The sun damage can be largely prevented, as I've previously stated, by wearing Chap

Stick *15-rated* Lip Balm. Another great one is Eclipse Lip Protectant.

Q: Are the chemicals used in sunscreens safe to use on babies and children?

A: Absolutely! In fact that's exactly when they should be started. If you'll put sunscreening lotion on your kids with each sun exposure, you'll be doing them a favor ranking right up there with love and a good education. You just can't start too early.

DERMALERT

Babies get sun damage as easily, if not more easily, than adults. They need sunscreens possibly even more than we do.

Q: My face burns up even with the use of a hat. Must I wear a sunscreen as well? Why?

A: A hat goes a long way toward preserving your beautiful unwrinkled complexion, but *reflected* sun is the real culprit for you. As much as 90 percent of the incident sunlight on sand can come shooting right back in your face. There's even *more* reflectance around water. Even *grass* reflects about 18 percent of the light that strikes it. So don't expect your hat to do it all. Use a sunscreening lotion as well.

DERMALERT

Reflected sun can sizzle your skin even faster than direct sunlight. Consider this when you're outside around water, white sand, or any highly reflectant surface.

PABA Allergy

Q: What do you do if you're allergic to sunscreen products?

A: The most common allergy to sunscreen products is, unfortunately, to the most effective ingredient, PABA. When this allergy occurs, the light-exposed areas break out in a rash of small bumps that itch like crazy. Without treatment, they last for days, and then fade slowly.

It's a tough problem, because PABA's so effective. However, the makers of sunscreens have come up with non-PABA-containing lotions, such as the new Solbar PF. This sunscreen should work wonders for those who couldn't wear sunscreens previously, because of allergies.

Q: Is PABA, taken orally, effective against sunburn, or is it more effective as a lotion?

A: PABA, taken internally in the form of Potaba tablets for severe skin diseases such as scleroderma, is a help, occasionally, in those diseases. But no evidence has ever been brought to my attention that it works at all as an "internal sunscreen."

Tanning Pills, Lotions, and Stains

Q: What are the yellow pills now being sold over the counter to those who like the "tanned look" in Canada and Europe?

A: These pills are made up of a substance called *canthaxanthin* which stains the skin a peculiar tan-yellow color. This so-called sunless tan is really quite weird looking, and I don't expect that the pills will go over very well here in the United States when they are released.

One big drawback, assuming that the tan they give looks natural, and that they're harmless, is that they stain the skin from below, without having any intrinsic sunscreening action. A person who is ordinarily quite cautious about the sun until a deep protective tan is obtained, might mistakenly sunbathe not realizing that he or she actually has no protection whatsoever. This could result in a lot of painful burns.

DERMALERT

Tanning pills, known as canthaxanthins, will have no protectant effect for the skin in sunlight.

Q: What are the side effects, if any, of taking Oxsoralen, a suntanning product?

A: The class of drugs called *psoralens* are terrific photosen-sitizers, that is, they induce a much exaggerated response to sun-light. Tanning with Oxsoralen occurs very quickly and with much deeper color. Psoralens are capable of inducing severe sunburns, however, and have done this to unwary sunbathers. While Oxsor-alen is extremely effective in clearing psoriasis, the risk of severe burns, eye problems, skin cancers, and other difficulties is suf-ficient enough to keep me from ever experimenting with it, except in the worst of skin disease-affected patients.

Q: Are the "quick-tanning" products safe? I apply the tan-ning cream to my skin. What are they made of?

A: In general, these temporary skin stains are safe, although I've seen an occasional allergic reaction to them. If you get any rashes while using them, just keep the products in mind as pos-sible causes. According to the Drug Information Center at the University of Kentucky, dihydroxyacetone, which is a form of dye, is the major substance in most quick-tanning products, and is known to be a substance that "tans without the sun."

Sunburn

Q: What can be done for severe sunburn in order to make movement easier?

A: That really depends on *how* severe it is. There are two common degrees of sunburn. I'll review the treatments of each type.

First-degree burn is that which just causes redness of the skin. It heals spontaneously over a few days, usually with desqua-mation, that is, the peeling of the upper layer of the epidermis, which is shed after the damage is repaired. It's painful, and the best treatments are topical and internal cortisones, which can calm the stinging and redness quite fast. Aspirin, as quickly as possible after you know you're burned, is a great help. Some experts think aspirin is good to take even *before* you incur the burn, because it's been discovered that aspirin inhibits an inflammation-causing compound called *prostaglandin*, which seems to cause the redness.

DERMALERT

If you know you are going to be in the sun for an extended time and cannot get a sunscreen, aspirin may help you control the damage done to your skin.

Redness results from damage to the tiny skin capillaries, which swell up massively when the sun irritates them. I've seen sunburn so severe that the capillaries have even leaked out tiny dots of blood below the skin!

Second-degree sunburn consists of blisters. It can be a true medical emergency if a large enough area is affected. It's very important to treat this as soon as possible because fluid loss can occur. This can cause weakness and even shock if severe enough.

Treatment includes steroids, both topically and internally, as well as cool soaks, antibiotics, and sometimes even tetanus reimmunization. *Every* second-degree blistering sunburn should be seen and treated by a doctor.

Q: I am 78 years old, and when I get in the sun, my face gets as red as blood and burns all over. I love to work outside on my flower garden, and every year I try to go on vacation with my daughter and son-in-law, but it is getting tough. Traveling is not very pleasant when the sun is shining. If you can help me with this, I would appreciate it.

A: When I read your letter, the first thing I wanted to know was if you are taking any medicines. That's because medicines often are a cause of your problem, which is photodermatitis. For instance, medicines such as the thiazide diuretics ("water pills"), which, in your age group are quite commonly used to control high blood pressure and the leg swelling which can result from bad leg circulation and heart failure, can cause a violent stinging, redness, burning, and itchy skin rash.

The next most frequent cause of photodermatitis is soap. Harsh antibacterial soaps can and do quite often cause the reaction to the sun of which you speak. That's because they contain an antibiotic substance that reacts with the sunlight.

DERMALERT

Medicines such as diuretics, antidiabetic agents, tranquilizers, antibiotics, and certain soaps can cause violent sun allergies.

Of course, there are many other causes of this sun stinging reaction, and your dermatologist will undoubtedly take a detailed history to determine the exact cause.

Get Sunglasses—Big Ones!

Q: What's a good type of protective sunglasses?

A: My favorites are Fisherman's Sunglasses, from the Orvis Company. They're polarized, with eye protection shields above and at the sides of the eyes. The Noir sunglasses, built originally for skiers and for patients who must undergo powerful light therapy for psoriasis, are good too. You can get them through:

Elder Pharmaceuticals, Inc.
705 East Mulberry Street
Bryan, Ohio 43506

Moles (Nevi)

Q: What's the difference between a wart and a mole?

A: The following chart will tell you the principal differences. But if you have *any* doubt, see your dermatologist!

Q: What causes hair to grow on moles? Can I remove it with tweezers? I'm a senior citizen and I've been wondering about these ugly hairs for years.

A: Moles form deep down in the skin, at the level of the formation of the hair follicles. The dark hairs and the moles develop together. I've had many patients come into the office complaining that they are tired of clipping off the hairs over their moles.

CHARACTERISTICS OF WARTS, MOLES, AND MELANOMAS

CHARACTERISTIC	WART	MOLE	MELANOMA
Color	Pale, skin-colored	Varied (pale, tan, brown, black)	Brown-black + red, white, or blue
Surface	Rough	Smooth to bumpy	Smooth to crusted and bleeding
Border	Even	Mostly even to uneven	Irregular, notched
Grouped	Yes, often	Very rarely	No
Infectious	Yes, virus-caused	No	No
Genetic predisposition	No	Yes	Occasionally
Malignant potential	None or very rare	Occasional but rare	These *are* malignant
Location	Hands, feet most common	Chest, back, face, scalp most common	Anywhere
Blackened surface capillaries	Yes	No	No, but may bleed intermittently
Congenital (present at birth)	No	Occasional	Rarely
Influenced by sunburns	No	No	Yes

"Why aren't you just plucking them out?" I usually ask.

"Why Dr. Bark," they ask agitatedly, "didn't you know that'll cause skin cancer in them?"

"As a matter of fact, I didn't! Where'd you hear that, anyway?"

"My Granny said a relative of her aunt's mother pulled a hair out of a black mole and she died of cancer."

"Hmmm. Sounds like really accurate firsthand information,

doesn't it? Just remember that you can believe only 50 percent of what you read, and 0 percent of what you hear, okay?"

DERMALERT

It's okay to pull the hairs out of a mole.

The fact is that these hairs have nothing to do with the malignant potential of moles. Moles are just collections of pigment-containing cells, and they have no more tendency to turn into skin cancers than any pigment cell anywhere in the body—and there are millions of them! The majority of melanoma skin cancers (the "deadly" type) arise *de novo*, i.e., in spots where absolutely no mole ever existed. Other melanomas, which the patient thinks arose from a mole, were already skin cancer from day one. But their slow growth in one location makes them look as though they were originally just moles. So go ahead and pull all the hairs out of your moles if you wish.

Q: Would accidentally scraping off a mole be dangerous?

A: Patients always want to know about the effect of irritation on moles. In short, it's not likely to produce a skin cancer that wasn't there already, but the fact that you tend to scrape this one off in your daily activities may mean that you should, in fact, consider having it removed to avert this concern in the future. I would.

Q: I have a small mole on my scalp, and my doctor says he wants to do something called a shave biopsy. Will my hair be gone in the spot where he removes it? Will it return?

A: Most dermatologists remove moles by this shave biopsy technique. In this method of removal, the mole is anesthetized with a tiny drop of medicine. This allows a painless procedure without distortion of the mole's surface. Then the mole is removed so that it is level with the surrounding skin. It's called a "shave biopsy" as opposed to an incisional biopsy, in which the lesion is cut full thickness out of the skin. In most cases, the incisional biopsy needs sutures, whereas the shave biopsy does not. Scarring and healing time are usually minimal with the shave technique. A nice smooth result is usually obtained in this manner. Note that moles are, for the most part, located deep down in the dermis, and therefore, for most moles, only the major fraction is removed by this technique. But it's enough to get a flat-looking spot where there used to be a bump, and a diagnosis is obtained on the biopsy specimen so obtained.

In the old days, doctors used to burn them off with electric needles, or just cut them off and throw them away. These methods are definitely to be condemned, because they don't allow for the sending off of the specimen to be checked by a pathologist for any possible signs of skin cancer. *Make sure that anything removed from your body is sent to a pathologist for examination.* Otherwise you can never know the exact kinds of cells which made up your mole.

The hair exactly over your mole will be removed for the shave biopsy procedure, but it grows back rapidly. Your dermatologist will tell you that since, in this method of removal, there are often some mole cells left, there is at least some chance that the mole could regrow, causing a new molelike bump which may need to be re-treated.

Q: I have a mole on my left shoulder that got sunburned this past summer. Now I have a white ring around the darker mole. Is this skin cancer?

A: Although I'd like to tell you that the sunburn activated the change in the mole to create the halo around it, I cannot. This is a fairly classic description of a mole called *Sutton's nevus,* or *halo nevus.* This strange reaction in a mole is just one more way that the body's fabulous immune system is able to patrol for problems inside our bodies.

It's apparent that some change is occurring inside the mole which has prompted the immune system to send out the body's defenses to wipe out the problem area. Many dermatologists feel these halo nevi are the precursors to true melanomas, the deadly pigmented skin cancers. Often, melanoma patients will develop halos around their normal moles, which can mean that they are fighting off their melanoma with greater success.

DERMALERT

If a whitish halo develops around a mole, have the mole taken off.

While most of us do shave biopsy these halo nevi, I have never yet seen a melanoma develop in one. So maybe the changes are so early as to be indistinguishable under the pathologist's microscope. Some clinicians choose to just watch these moles, but, following the golden rule, I can only say that I'd want my *own* Sutton's nevus off if I developed one, so I can do no less for my patients.

Proof that this halo represents the elimination of the mole comes from patients with *just* the halo, having absolutely no mole left whatsoever! They'll often say that they've noticed the disappearance of a large mole that was there several months ago. Strange! And sometimes, the pigment returns to its normal color.

While it's not possible to say that the damaging rays of the sun actually caused your individual problem, we know from extensive studies in Australia that even a single severe sunburn is associated with a marked increase in the incidence of malignant melanoma. The importance of this is obvious. If you can keep your kids out of severe sun, just think what a greater chance they'll have to grow up "skin cancer-free."

Q: I have a mole which I have had on my back for some time. It is soft in nature, but it seems to have another mole growing on top of it! It itches very badly sometimes. I see now that it has a white ring around it. Should this be removed or not?

A: Get it off yesterday! You've already got three of the cardinal signs of skin cancer: pigmentary change, growth change, and, most important, *itching!* Even though those soft, fleshy moles such as yours seldom, if ever, turn into skin cancer, the fact is that if it *is* a cancer, the statistics are 100 percent in your case. Can you afford to take that chance? Absolutely not!

DERMALERT

Any growth in a mole may be an indicator that a skin cancer is developing.

Q: Is there any research going on about what causes moles and what can be done to prevent them? What possibility is there that lasers will begin to be used to remove moles as they are now used to remove birthmarks?

A: There's plenty of ongoing research about moles, but most of it has been centered not on the cause (which is assumed to be genetic) but on their accidental relationship to skin cancers, which I've already discussed.

There appears to be very little probability that lasers will be used for the primary removal of moles. Lasers cut with a beam of light which is at least as hot as the *sun*, and this intense burning precludes the proper analysis of the cells of the specimen to be removed, by far the most important thing in removing your mole.

Q: Is there any kind of cream I can buy to cover up a very dark, black, irregular spot on my cheek? The older I get the more weird spots I see. I have been using a skin bleach for several years, but it does not really seem to help. I hope you can tell me about a cream that I can use, so I won't have to go to the doctor.

A: Go to your doctor immediately. The description of your cheek spot fits that of a type of premalignant or malignant spot called *lentigo maligna.* This type of spot should be seen *as soon as it appears*, because a malignant melanoma may be present.

Too many people have a propensity to self-treat skin diseases for far too long. If you treat a spot with an over-the-counter medicine and it doesn't clear promptly, you *must* have it checked. I just hope yours hasn't progressed too far already.

Q: I have a *real* mole problem. On my chest, above the breast, I have a two-inch-square area containing, believe it or not, about 100 very tiny moles! They've been there since my birth, and I was wondering what you'd think would be the best form of removal.

A: It sounds as if you have a type of congenital "mosaic" nevus. That's a pigmented mole which is formed of many parts. If it has indeed been present since your birth, you should have it removed, because current statistics show that 10 to 17 percent of these lesions turn into a particularly vicious form of malignant melanoma. I've discussed this in Chapter 3, so you ought to reread the section on congenital nevi.

Usually, excisional surgery is needed to remove them so that
no regrowth is likely. This can be done either by a plastic surgeon
or by a dermatologist.

What to Do If You Suspect Skin Cancer

Q: I believe that I have a skin cancer on my ear. There is
a black scablike spot on the upper section of my left ear, and I
am greatly concerned about it. Several times this scab has dropped
off. However, this has not occurred for several months. What
should I do?

A: This is a classic presentation and location for a sun cancer
and, as I often say, you should *run*, not walk, to your dermatologist. It sounds as though something definitely has happened in
your skin to make healing difficult, and any nonhealing sore
should be checked as soon as possible. Probably a biopsy will
be done to examine the tissue for microscopic signs of a skin
cancer.

Q: My problem is eczema. I have an embarrassing red mark
the size of a penny on my arm, plus a couple of other inconspicuous marks. They don't bother me but they sure don't look very
nice. My doctor tells me there is nothing that can be done for
them. Is this true?

A: Probably not. Your question is important because of your
probably mistaken assumption that your skin problem is eczema.
This happens so often in dermatology that it's frankly tragic. Patients should not be *diagnosing* problems, they should just be
spotting them. That is, you really don't have the training to tell
the exact nature of most skin lesions. If your assumption that
you've got eczema is wrong, you could *die* for the mistake! Just
remember that any scaly spot which stays in one place could be
a premalignant or malignant lesion. In good conscience, you've
just got to have it checked. Don't forget, the person who plays
doctor and "treats himself has a fool for a patient!"

How about the doctor who said nothing could be done? Unfortunately, while all dermatologists are doctors, the reverse is
not true. One cannot be expected to know every form of therapy

for every possible skin disease, plus all the facts necessary to be a general medical doctor too. We only hope that books like this can aid the lay public and help the individual fill in the gaps in some way.

DERMALERT

When you notice a skin problem, don't try to diagnose it. Your job is over once you've spotted the problem. Get a *dermatologist* to make the correct diagnosis.

Q: My husband has had skin cancer (from sun exposure) removed from his upper ears. He now has an area of blotches on his upper cheeks and uses old-fashioned zinc oxide to keep the sun out. But this only protects the skin when he is outside working, and I am worried about all the sun he has received in the *past*. What can he do about all that past damage?

A: As I said earlier in this chapter, the constant bombardment of the radiation of the sun builds up and remains over a person's entire lifetime. He'll never, in short, get rid of the tendency to have sunspots and skin cancers. In fact, we have to watch patients who have had one or more skin cancers removed for the development of new ones over subsequent years. Statistics show that these folks are prone to getting more cancers.

Q: Does sunlight cause internal cancers too?

A: Not that anyone is aware of. That is, unless you'd count the internal spread of sun-induced skin cancers, such as melanoma.

Sun Freckles

Q: What causes the brown spots on the skin when I lie in the sun? What can be done about them?

A: These flat, usually nonscaly brown spots, often found on the sides of the face and elsewhere, are called *actinic lentigo* or sun freckles. Sometimes they have an element of AK in them. They are removed beautifully by light cryosurgery. They darken with continued sun exposure, so protect them from sunlight if at all possible.

I certainly hope in this chapter you've learned something about sun cancer, moles, melanoma, and the proper care of your skin in the sun. As the American Cancer Society says, "Use *sense* in the sun!"

18

Herpes—The New Leprosy

A man walked up to a waiter and asked, "May I please trouble you for a glass of water, sir?"

A woman behind a table, usually of good nature, glanced at the horrible weeping sores on his face and exclaimed, "Don't serve his kind anything! We don't want *them* around here!"

What a terrible disease leprosy can be! But wait. Not leprosy, you say? Of course not. It's a modern scene in any *singles bar* in our land! And unfortunately, it happens not once, but thousands of times daily to the unfortunate victims of the herpes simplex virus (HSV).

But why? Why, in this land of modern medical miracles of every imaginable sort, are we completely unable to shut off this terrible disease? Where did this terrible scourge come from anyway? Is there *nothing* we can do? Must we suffer this malady forever?

In this chapter, I'd like to examine the myths and madness surrounding the herpes controversy, from the standpoint of one who treats patients with HSV every day. I'll try to answer the common and uncommon questions about the disease, and tell you exactly how *I* treat herpes of various types for my own patients, right in my office.

First, I should mention that for all the television shows, specials, and guest appearances I've done on the subject of HSV, I've gotten remarkably little mail asking questions about it. I've tried to imagine why this might be. At first I thought that the public was fed up with hearing about this incurable disease. But whenever we do a television show in the "call-in" format, the switchboards are swamped with calls. That led me to the real understanding of why more questions about the HSV aren't asked. Actually, *Time* magazine tipped me off to the possible solution about a year ago, with their detailed, excellent cover story on the national disaster of HSV.

The August 2, 1982 edition of *Time* stated, in an aside to the cover story, that they had had a devil of a time finding models to pose for the front cover! This normally quite lucrative assignment went *begging* for models willing to be identified with the "scourge" of HSV. In short, people don't want to be identified in any way, shape, or form with the thought that they might have the dreaded disease. Even patients who are forced by the condition to seek treatment at my office are extremely reluctant to discuss their real problem.

Psychiatrists tell me that they're often consulted by patients who found it impossible to relate normally after contracting herpes. They say the victims feel "unclean" and "untouchable," just like the lepers of ancient times. But just as today's victims of true leprosy live in fair comfort in society, it's possible for the herpes patient to make his or her way successfully through social situations. Note that I didn't say *easy*, just *possible*.

Since there are two common presentations of herpes simplex, I've chosen to talk about the most common form, oral herpes, first.

Cold Sores

Q: Every time I get too much sun, my lips break out in fever blisters. Someone told me if I took vitamin B every day and used a sunscreen, I'd be all right. Are they right?

A: Oral herpes simplex is also known as fever blisters, cold sores, and "sun poisoning." Actually, that tells you a lot about what activates them. But where'd you get them in the first place, and why do they keep coming back? To understand your enemy may not, in this case, be to conquer, but it'll sure help.

The herpes virus is the ultimate parasite. It's a tiny DNA virus; that is, it has the very stuff of life, DNA, as its core. The virus probably hits us all at one time or another, but some of us are infected and some are not. Why? Unhappily, that's one of the numerous less-than-well-understood facts about this incredible organism. Some think since the virus lives *inside* the cell, that the normal antibodies which defend us in similar situations cannot reach the virus inside the cell to kill it.

But which cells does the virus ordinarily live in? It actually maintains its home in the ganglia, or nerve clusters, that emanate from the spinal cord and brain. So it's a nerve-infecting virus. To reinfect the skin with a new set of blisters, it must travel down the skin nerves and out onto the skin, where it again invades the cells of the skin itself.

There the virus activates and starts to reproduce its genetic material, thus making new virus particles. When this happens, the cells which had been previously infected with the herpes virus are burst open, or lysed, killing them and releasing thousands of virus particles into the surrounding area. It's during this time that the virus (and the rash it obviously causes) is spread to adjacent cells.

Once the new cells are parasitized by the virus, the whole process starts again. In this way, infection with the virus is per-petuated—infection after painful, irritated, blistering infection. This very complicated replication process is one of the main areas in which research is being conducted to find a cure for herpes.

So sunlight activates your herpes sores? Join the club. It's probably the infection's most common aggravant. My office floods with herpes patients after every sunny, home football game at the University of Kentucky here in Lexington. Why it happens is not that clear, but it appears that the damaging rays of the sun, which we dermatologists decry so often, stun the defenses of the skin cells in which the virus lives, thus allowing the virus to begin to multiply. The same mechanism is obviously at work for febrile illnesses (those with fevers) and, so the majority of dermatologists feel, in times of great emotional stress. Although those of us who consider ourselves "scientific dermatologists" like to think that no skin diseases are caused by emotions, it's really hard to stick to that opinion when patient after patient says that emotions bring on the attacks.

Vitamin B is completely worthless for fighting fever blister attacks. Its use is just another example of how laypeople, when they don't know what to do for a skin disease, turn to the only thing they *can* control, diet and vitamins. Don't waste your time. Sunscreens are another story, however. They help by shielding the delicate skin cells from the sun's radiation. Without sun, the virus is not encouraged to multiply. Good sunscreens for this purpose include heavy opaque lipsticks, Chap Stick Sunblock 15 Lip Balm, and Eclipse Lip Protectant.

Don't forget the age-old trick of wearing a broad-brimmed hat while you're outside. And try, if you can, to sit on the *shady* side of the stadium, or in a seat in partial shade anywhere.

Q: But where the heck did *I* get herpes in the first place?

A: When you were an infant, some careless, unknowing adult with a big, juicy herpes simplex sore on his or her lips scooped you up off the floor and planted a huge, wet, virus-laden smooch right on your lips exactly in the place where you now have your recurrent herpes simplex lesions. Disgusting! But it's a good lesson for all of us to remember—if you've got oral herpes simplex sores, you've absolutely no place around babies, infants, toddlers, or anybody else who doesn't especially want a lifetime of painful, weeping, oozing lip sores.

Q: Is there any difference between a cold sore and a fever blister?

A: No. Each name just tells you the possible activator of the disease in an individual case. Colds, fever, stress, sunlight, and extreme fatigue are said to be initiators of the blisters.

Genital HSV

Q: What is genital type II herpes simplex?

A: The herpes simplex viruses are generally divided into type I and type II. Type I was generally felt to be the type which attacked the lips, and type II was supposed to be the type that struck the genitalia. This division is a lot less useful today, because both types are found in both regions. This is thought to be a result of the changing sexual mores in this country which permit oral-genital sexual contact. This form of sex is directly responsible for the transference of the virus to the "new" areas where it had not previously been a frequent resident.

Q: Is type II herpes harder to treat?

A: In general, yes. It's a tougher virus, and doesn't respond very well to the soothing treatments we usually use in the disease. We'll talk a lot more about treatment in a minute.

Q: Genital herpes—could it look like a cluster of warts?

A: Nope! Herpes is a *blistering* disease, first, last and in between. It may ulcerate, or break down to weeping sores, from time to time, but look like warts it doesn't! Warts are warts; herpes is herpes. But remember that they can both be considered to be venereal diseases, and they're both very communicable, so *get yourself treated*!

Q: What's the fatality rate of herpes type II?

A: Rarely will a victim of primary (i.e., first infection) herpes simplex develop encephalitis, or brain infection, with the virus. While this is an extremely rare event, it's also extremely fatal. Most of these patients die. Some of the newer drugs we'll discuss later may help them survive.

Q: I develop a fever about twelve hours before I get vulvar HSV. Then I get tingling spots on my labia which break out shortly in blisters. Is the fever common?

A: We call this the *viral prodrome*, or warning signal that a new attack is coming. Many patients feel peculiar prior to the onset of the skin lesions, and can very accurately predict that they'll have a new crop of painful blisters in a day or two. Maybe it's the fever that tips them off. I don't know of any good studies to show what causes them to know that they'll break out, but many do.

Of course, the first-time victim often has a much more severe course than the patient with a subsequent attack.

A Plausible Theory

Q: My daughter had a breakout on her lower spine after a prolonged labor with her first child. It was diagnosed as herpes, brought on by stress. Since we know it's a contagious virus, our whole family is worried about the possibility of its passing from one person to another. Can the spread be stopped?

A: Certainly the strain of a difficult delivery can result in the activation of a new crop of herpes blisters. That's most assuredly why your daughter got her new episode. Certainly herpes is a contagious disease and therefore can be transmitted. But there is little or no chance that other family members could get the disease from her. In order to do this, it would be necessary to touch the spot where the disease occurs, or she would have to touch the spot and then immediately touch another person with some of the wet exudate (fluid from the blisters) on her hands. Both these possibilities would have to be considered unlikely if the barest minimum of precautions are taken, such as simple hand washing. In short, the family need not worry. But you should become acquainted with some of the other reasons why people get the disease on their buttocks.

Recently, in the *Schoch Letter*, a respected monthly newsletter circulated to every dermatologist in the country, a couple of explanations were proposed for why women contract buttock herpes. One of these is that they sit down on strange toilet seats from time to time, thus picking up the virus in a very logical place— that part of their anatomy which contacts the seat. It is thought that the virus *does* actually live a short time on the seat after it has been deposited, and infects its new host with great relish. At some time in the near future, then, the newly infected woman sits down with an active sore on *her* buttock, and unwittingly adds another statistic to the crowded rolls of herpes sufferers.

The other proposed explanation is, in my mind, even more

plausible. It's called "spooning."[1] After a man and woman complete sexual intercourse, the woman, because of her usually somewhat smaller stature, often rolls over with her back toward her mate, and he cuddles close to her, facing her backside. It's like two "spoons" fitting into one another. If he has a herpes sore on his penis, he drips virus onto her buttock for some time thereafter. Voilà! A new herpes patient. It's a sad but highly probable explanation for this type of herpes in women.

More on Contagion

Q: I have had herpes simplex on my sacrum for several months. I have been under the care of a dermatologist who has been treating me with amino acid tablets. It seems to be helping. I noticed the problem after a fall on my tailbone some time ago. Do you have any patients like me?

A: Far too many of them! In fact, I'm convinced that trauma plays a larger role in the development of herpes than previously thought. I have one patient, a notable athlete, who never had herpes prior to irritating his rear and sacral area doing strenuous sit-ups in a strange motel. Because he was anxious to stay in peak condition, he had done a tremendous number of sit-ups in nothing but an athletic supporter! The long "shag" carpet in the motel must have eroded away the protective dead layer of the skin just enough to embed the virus, and start his lifetime infection with herpes simplex.

Q: Can I get herpes from a swimming pool?

A: Probably not. The chlorine in the pool kills the virus rapidly.

The Lysine Controversy

Q: I am writing to ask the name of the drug used to treat

---

[1] Schoch Letter, Volume 34, Number 2, February 1984.

herpes sores. I did not catch the whole name, but it began with an "L." Why is there not a cure for herpes?

A: Before getting into this all-important area, let me tell you a fascinating story. Several years ago some researchers growing herpesvirus in culture allowed the concentration of one crucial ingredient to get too high, thus killing off all the valuable viral cultures in their laboratory. Disappointed at first, elation overcame them as they realized what they had discovered. The ingredient, L-lysine, had just *killed off* the herpes virus!

L-Lysine is a harmless amino acid, a necessary building block in the construction of thousands of proteins in the human body. Why not, the scientists reasoned, load a person with herpes simplex full of the compound and see what happens to the disease? The stuff's taken into the body, and any excess is eventually used or excreted, so little harm could be done. Well, it worked! In the first tests, many patients seemed to get well faster and not get recurrences as often.

Subsequent tests in very carefully controlled studies, however, showed that there was essentially no effect on the virus or the disease. My problem with these later studies is that the researchers employed very low doses of the L-Lysine. In practice, my patients tell me that they do much better with their herpes when they are taking fairly massive doses of say, three to six grams (3,000 to 6,000 milligrams) per day. At this range, patients claim to get better faster, and, if they continue to take L-lysine after the attack, tend to get fewer recurrences (and milder ones) at later dates.

The stuff is worth a try. If it doesn't work, then give it up. Complications are just about nil. I've had one patient who got diarrhea on it, but otherwise, I've seen virtually no problems. One note of caution. The human body will only use L-lysine, not the D-form. To be sure that you're getting the right stuff, make sure that you only get the brand Enisyl (that's "Lysine" spelled backwards).

Since you asked about prevention, I'll mention a little about it as far as L-lysine is concerned. In the dosage range of five to six 500-milligram tablets per day, most of my patients say they have far fewer, and less severe, attacks. And if a lesion does appear, they increase the dosage at the first possible instant they recognize the symptoms of a new attack.

Why not a cure? Because the herpesvirus is a tough little critter to get our immunologic hands on. It "lives" *inside* the cell, where our magnificent antibodies can't go. And after years of research, we're just now beginning to develop drugs active against viruses without damaging the vital biochemical machinery in the cytoplasm and nucleus of human cells. I'll mention one such miracle drug shortly.

Other Treatments

Q: What else is available to treat this terrible problem?

A: For thousands of years, hot soaks have been used to ease the pain of the acute herpes infection. I usually suggest that my patients soak the affected area several times daily with very warm (*not* burning!) tap water on a washcloth. This seems to decrease the swelling and tenderness of the acute eruption.

Other drying agents, such as ether (explosive), acetone (flammable), and alcohol (ineffective *and* flammable) were tried and found to be almost as good as *hoping* the herpes would go away.

Zovirax

Q: In the early summer, I tend to develop herpes on my face. What's the best thing to do when it first develops?

A: Besides the L-lysine we already discussed, you should know about a new antiviral ointment for herpes, called *acyclovir* (brand name Zovirax). Invented by researchers at the Burroughs Wellcome Company, it is one of the cleverest drugs ever devised. This substance kills the virus, but only after the virus itself *activates* the drug! They've actually enlisted the infection to help kill itself off!

But there's bad news along with the good news about acyclovir. First the good news—in primary herpes simplex sufferers, the drug lessens symptoms, shortens the time of viral shedding, and promotes healing, when the ointment is applied every three hours, six times daily. Now for the bad news—it's *not* useful in recurrent herpes sufferers, except to decrease the duration of shedding of the infectious virus. For all practical purposes, that pretty well kills it as a practical drug for the average repeatedly infected patient.

But don't lose all hope because of the apparent ineffectiveness of acyclovir ointment in recurrent disease. A new form may be taken orally. The capsule form is taken five times daily at the first sign of an attack. They are continued for five days per attack, and have several advantages over the ointment. First, the capsules *do* appear to shorten the morbidity (pain and associated symptoms) and time course of the infection. The virus cannot usually be cultured from the lesions after taking the medicine for only twenty-four hours.

Currently the medicine is FDA-approved for use in only genital herpes simplex. It may also be used as a preventive, in doses of three capsules daily, for up to six months. Again, this medicine is not a *cure*, but it's by far the best drug ever developed for HSV.

An intravenous form already on the market apparently helps those who develop generalized herpes simplex. This disease usually afflicts patients who are very ill due to some other serious cause, such as lymphoma or other types of cancer, or else immunosuppressed because of a transplant of some kind.

Another problem with acyclovir is the development of resistance by the virus to it. This could be a very drastic consequence; since the virus is "smart" enough to skirt the drug (as some variants of herpes simplex do with acyclovir), this may severely limit the drug's usefulness in the treatment of common herpes simplex.

Q: I have HSV on the left side of my nose. It recurs every three to six months with a duration of about *six weeks!* During this time I have had a bandage on my nose all the time to cover this nickel-sized sore. The reason I'm writing you is to ask what type of surgery can be done to resolve herpes simplex, such as removal of the nerves in that area of the nose. Or do you know of any experimental drug programs that can deal with this?

A: Six weeks is an excessive length of time, even for a severe case, and I'd suspect that you might be promoting a bacterial infection by keeping the sore covered with an adhesive bandage. That's what those things do best, you know. Throw the bandages in the trash can and let the spot heal normally, taking the precautions we've already mentioned in this chapter. Remember that Zovirax may really help a person such as yourself, who has really severe attacks.

Surgery? It won't help. The nervous system is pretty smart. It'll just regrow the tiny nerve twigs into the skin where they've been surgically removed, and you'll get herpes, possibly *worse* herpes, in the scar. There is no surgery which will help this disease. In fact, neurosurgeons discovered early on that herpes is a neurotrophic (nerve-infecting) virus when they noticed outbreaks of the disease after operating on the ganglia, or nerve clumps, which supply the face.

There are experimental drug programs for herpes simplex all over the country. You would do best to contact your local medical school or their department of dermatology. They'll know what research is being done in your area.

Above all, get that nose sore *checked* by a dermatologist. It could be an early skin cancer or any number of other problems you may not have recognized.

Q: I've always wanted to know how a dermatologist would behave if he or she were single in this society. Would he or she go to singles bars, date, and so forth, knowing about the diseases that could be caught?

A: A common joke these days in dermatologic circles is that you can always tell who the dermatologist is in the restroom—the one who washes his or her hands *before* going to the bathroom! While of course it's right to worry about contagion these days, with all the strange venereal diseases going around, one cannot let that fear be totally occupying. However, most dermatologists I know would be extraordinarily careful to avoid multiple sexual contacts. I guess the old monogamous ways were indeed the best from the standpoint of venereal diseases. I hate to sound puritanical, but it becomes obvious that multiple contacts increase the chances of getting these contagious diseases exponentially. On many occasions, I've seen college kids come in with *three* or *four* venereal diseases *at once*.

Until the cures for the viral venereal diseases such as herpes simplex are found, sexual relationships must be handled the same way porcupines make love—very carefully. Get to know your prospective partner. Don't bed down with anyone who appears to be in pain, or has sores of any kind *anywhere*. Do not have oral sex with anyone who has lip sores, swellings, or fever blisters. *Ask* your prospective partner if he or she has any communicable diseases such as herpes, gonorrhea, syphilis, warts, or molluscum. Certainly not everyone is completely honest, but believe it or not, some still are. And use condoms; they may protect you from not only the herpes infection but also from many other venereal diseases.

Not long ago, I saw a personal ad for a person with herpes looking to date another who also had the disease! Sounds like a bright idea, doesn't it, until you realize that you could be contracting another strain of HSV or getting it in an area where you never had it before. It's a terrible situation our sex-oriented society is in. The search goes on each day for a new compound which will finally put to rest the "new leprosy," but it hasn't yet been found. Perhaps chemists, vaccine researchers, and dermatologists will find ways to prevent the spread of HSV in the near future, but for now, limiting contacts, investigating them, and frank discussion of sexually transmitted diseases are the only ways available to someone trying to live a disease-free existence.

Recent studies show that the HSV can be cultured from the skin even when the actual sores are *not* present. This makes the "swinging single" life even that more complicated. The bottom line appears to be: Do your thing, if you must, but do it carefully, and with your eyes wide open to the possible consequences.

19

Winter Itch—The Problems of Dry Skin

It was another freezing January day in Lexington. Winter was taking its usual heavy toll on skin. My first patient of the day was bent over, scratching and digging at her legs.

"Dr. Bark, you've got to help me," said the frustrated woman patient. "My family has threatened to move me into the basement if I don't quit scratching my legs!" She pulled up a pant leg to reveal a shin loaded with tiny bleeding cracks I recognized immediately as winter dry skin.

"How many times per day do you bathe?" I asked, anticipating her answer.

"Well, usually two, but the water makes my legs *feel* so good! It's later that they seem to itch so much."

"Aha! You've hit squarely on the problem. But you're really making the problem worse. Now let's see if a few modifications in your routine can improve your condition."

Winter after winter dermatologists hear such complaints of dry skin problems. And while dryness can strike any age group, it's much more common as one ages. It's really true that our oil gland output drops sharply after our teens. This decrease in oil-

271

iness plus winter dry air can lead straight to a case of severe dry skin.

But it's possible to live with smooth, supple skin even if you're not a teenager and even in winter. This chapter will teach you the secrets that dermatologists use to correct almost *any* dry skin problem.

Q: Can you recommend a lotion to calm the inflammation of my dry, irritated, scaly skin? Nothing has helped so far, and I'm ashamed to be seen. Can the lotion be used on my face also?

A: The condition you have is called *xerosis*. This is a term derived from a Greek word meaning "dryness." It should not be confused in name with psoriasis, the scaly red genetic skin disease, or cirrhosis, a disease of inflammation and hardening of the liver. (Psoriasis is discussed in detail in Chapter 16.) Xerosis is a very common, noninfectious disease which occurs with greater frequency during the fall and winter months because of the low humidity. In fact, many people call xerosis "winter itch" because during periods of low humidity, the skin dries out horribly. The condition is usually found in areas of the body where oil glands are not very numerous, such as the arms, legs, and trunk areas.

DERMALERT

Low humidity in the winter is one of the main causes of dry skin.

When the skin dries out, the dead top layer of the skin stiffens and cracks. This cracking causes fissures in the skin, which then become irritated, inflamed, and very itchy. This problem is by no means confined to one age group or sex. It is found in young children, as well as middle-aged and elderly adults. Even *teenagers* can get it on nonoily parts of their skin.

There are many contributing factors to xerosis besides the season of the year. The second most common cause is the usage of harsh antibacterial soaps. Some patients find that they contribute to dry skin. The newer liquid soaps in dispenser bottles are also extremely drying.

In fact, many of these soaps contain substances which, during the summer months, can even react with the sunlight striking the skin, causing an itchy eruption on the skin, which is very serious. We'll talk about the *right* soap to use in a minute.

The next most common cause of xerosis is excess bathing. Television and commercial advertisements have made us all too conscious of the "need" for frequent skin cleansing. Repeated washing removes the skin's natural oil layer. This allows evaporation of the skin's water, which, in turn, leaves the very substance of the skin dry. In other words, water and bathing are extremely *drying* to the skin! As a matter of fact, xerosis is only a product of recent years, because people never used to take as many baths as they do now, and if they only took one bath a week (whether they needed it or not), they had a chance to reaccumulate their natural body oils in between baths. Then they just didn't *have* dry skin.

DERMALERT

A bath a week may be plenty for a person with dry skin. In between baths, spot-bathe when you absolutely need to.

What can you do about your extremely dry skin? Decrease your baths to a maximum of one every other day, if possible. If you find it necessary to bathe in between your baths, just spot-bathe. Usually, Dove (recently found in two studies to be the mildest soap), used in small amounts, is perfectly adequate for cleansing. If you cannot use it for any reason, then use Emulave, Lowila, Basis, or Neutrogena soap.

The whole principle of bathing and soap use can be summed up by using the "three gits": "Git in, git clean, and git out!"

After bathing, it's absolutely crucial that you replace the oil you've washed off your skin. I prefer that you use a bath oil after each bath or shower, but do *not* follow the directions on the bottle. The instructions tell you to put the oil into the water. *Never put bath oil in your bath water!* This is wasteful because the bath oil, for the most part, goes down the drain instead of onto your skin.

The oil also makes the tub *extremely slippery*. So, to avoid both problems (losing most of your bath oil and slipping on it), you should apply the bath oil to your wet skin while standing *outside the tub*. You may then pat dry gently, but do not rub off the oil you've just applied.

DERMALERT

Bath oil should only be applied to your wet skin *after* your bath or shower.

Dry skin lotions have come a long way in 3,000 years, since the Egyptian women first used scented oils to coat their skin after bathing. That was really the first generation of moisturizers.

Second-generation moisturizers came along in the 1940s with the advent of oil-in-water emulsions. These moisturizers really just contained a lot of water and some oil to layer over the skin and seal in the water. This worked pretty well, but the skin still lost fantastic amounts of water through insensible loss, that is, the daily water evaporation of which none of us is aware.

In the 1970s, urea was added to the later second-generation moisturizers. Urea is a hygroscopic material, meaning it actually draws water into the skin and holds it there. The only trouble with urea was its tendency to sting when applied to tender areas of the skin.

That left the door open for the first of the third generation of moisturizers, Complex 15. This remarkable stuff, invented by the Baker/Cummins Division of the Key Pharmaceutical Company, contains a chemical derived from soybeans, called *lecithin*. Chemically, it's a phospholipid, which is a long molecule that can attract and hold up to fifteen molecules of water for every molecule of lecithin. And this vegetable derivative is so closely related to the skin's natural phospholipids that it won't even sting. As you might imagine, this is a tremendous advance over conventional moisturizers, with or without urea.

Actual experiments with living cells showed that when natural phospholipids were extracted they appeared to *die*, but when the active ingredient of Complex 15 was added, they came "back to life." That is, their chemistry seemed to start up again. If it will do this for animal cells, the hope is that it can keep our skin cells intact longer.

Some really amazing tests show how effective this stuff really is. In tests run in the dry, cold northeast, and the dry, super-hot southwest, volunteers applied Complex 15 to their extra-dry skin, and they cleared up their dryness immediately. The amazing thing is that they remained moist from the Complex 15 applications for up to ten days after they *stopped* using the lotion! That's how well phospholipids bind water into the skin! You can use it on your face with no problems. It even comes in a cream formulation, for those who prefer creams on their faces. If your pharmacy doesn't yet stock it, request that it be ordered, or you can write:

Baker/Cummins
Dermatological Division of Key Pharmaceuticals, Inc.
50 North West 176th Street
Miami, Florida 33169

Q: What about recommending something to use on my dry lips in the winter?

A: You have several options open to you for your lips in the winter. Most women who wear lipstick do just fine with only that, if they wear it regularly and reapply it often. But much better than lipstick is Eclipse Lip Protectant and Chap Stick. These have the obvious extra advantage of having excellent sunscreens contained within their formulations. They're especially good if you're going to be out in the snow in the wintertime, because the cold, dry air and intense sun damage can destroy soft lips quickly. Carbolated Vaseline is recommended by many allergists and dermatologists, but it's largely been supplanted by the lip protectants containing sunscreen.

DERMALERT

Even more important than the cold for your lips in winter is the effect of sun damage. Make sure you use a lip protectant with a sunscreen.

If you're not going to be outside much, regular Vaseline is an excellent product for restoring the necessary moisture to the lips. However, it's pretty easy to lick it off from time to time, so you'll have to concentrate on applying it frequently.

Q: You mentioned dry air as a cause of xerosis. Does that mean that a humidifier will help?

A: Yes, low humidity should be corrected if at all possible. This can be done quite adequately by obtaining a humidifier. The whole-house type, although more expensive, is the best because you can regulate your entire environment with the touch of a button. They'll commonly be able to increase the humidity to 45 to 50 percent, which should be sufficient to help your dry skin, assuming you're following my advice on bathing, soaps, bath oils, and so forth.

Another way, of course, is to buy the single-room type of humidifier. Be sure not to get a *de*humidifier, though. That could be disastrous. You might also consider leaving pans of water near heat duct openings, on radiators, and in other places. It even helps if you'll leave the commode lids open and leave a one-inch layer of water in the plugged bathtub all the time.

Q: What is the cause of nummular eczema? Is there a cure for it?

A: Nummular eczema is dry, scaly skin with coin-shaped patches. It's the most common form of winter itch on the arms and legs. Though actually a type of xerosis, it can be somewhat harder to clear, and you may need lotions containing cortisone to get it under control.

The spots begin as tiny circular patches which are most often said, by the patients and some of their referring doctors, to be ringworm. Antifungal creams don't have much effect, except to temporarily heal a patch or two, just because the medicine is slightly moisturizing.

Q: Is dry skin hereditary?

A: You bet! But it's hard to tell a person if he or she will get it or pass it on, because so many of us have dry skin anyway. In general, light-skinned, fair-haired, blue-eyed folks are dry-skinned, and dark-complected people are less dry.

Q: I read in a recent book on dry skin that we should all be *drinking* oil to help our dry skin! True?

A: Hogwash! The oil a person eats is broken down into its component parts just like any other food we eat. It never even reaches the skin as oil. So forget it.

Remember, if you take a few easy precautions against winter itch, you can make dry, cold weather a lot more tolerable. Moisturize, lubricate, virtually lather on the lotions during cool, dry weather, or whenever you itch, scale, and flake. You'll feel "cutaneously comfortable" if you do!

20

New Wrinkles on Aging Skin

Billions of dollars are spent each year in this country to try to reverse the effects of "TMB," or too many birthdays. Our youth-oriented society is immersed in the pursuit of the "young look," the "carefree look." Nothing strikes closer to the heart than to awaken one morning and look in the mirror to find a brown, scaly spot on your forehead—your very first "age spot"—staring right back at you. It's something that none of us feels will ever really happen to us, and it's all the more depressing when it does.

Not only do we not accept the signs of "advancing years" or "senior citizenry," but we swarm to the offices of dermatologists and plastic surgeons to seek redress, to have all traces of time erased. However, there are now terrific ways to seemingly reverse the years. They bring a famous skin researcher's saying several steps closer to reality: "The object of life is to die young, as late as possible."

In this chapter, I'll tell you about some problems of aging skin and how you and your dermatologist may stuff some of the sands of time back into the upper part of your hourglass. It's not completely a "do-it-yourself" chapter. My purpose here is to really *tell* you, for a change, what actually can be done for the signs of aging, and what results you should expect.

There's a huge number of problems accompanying aging skin. I've picked those which are most widely applicable, so that you can get an idea what types of procedures and medications are available to you.

The Pinch Test—The First Indicator

Q: I saw you demonstrate a "pinch test" to tell biological age. How does it work?

A: The pinch test is merely a demonstration of how much elasticity or stretchability is left in your skin. Try this: Just pinch up a fold of skin on the back of the hand, and then release it. In the teens and twenties, the skin snaps back instantly to its original contour. In the thirties and forties, it snaps back, but you can begin to see it stay up for a second before returning flat. That means that some of the skin's support network has changed as a result of age.

The really striking finding with the pinch test comes in the fifties, sixties, and seventies. Then the skin hangs up there for many seconds before returning to the flat. What's all this mean? It means that your whole body is undergoing this type of change, but the skin is the place where you can actually watch it happen.

Q: How does that guy at the carnival guess my age?

A: By being one heck of a good dermatologist! If you talk to them seriously, they will not very often be able to tell you the actual *way* they guess ages, but guess them they do! Actually, they take some real cutaneous clues from their "patients." First, they look at the state of wrinkling of the skin. That's why they hate to have blacks play the game. Their ages are *extremely* hard to guess because of the terrific sun protection they get from their natural sunscreen, melanin. (If you'll remember, that's the protective pigment in the epidermis which filters out the wrinkling rays of the sun. And without any wrinkles, the age guessing game is nearly impossible.)

There are other cutaneous clues, too, such as gray hair and

age spots. We'll be talking about many of these problems in this chapter.

Life's Barnacles—Seborrheic Keratoses

Q: I am a 59-year-old woman with very fair skin, but in the past few years, perhaps five or six, I have developed brownish-black blotches (moles?) on my back. They are becoming more numerous. They do not hurt or bother me, except during winter months. Then they itch slightly. Why do these develop in such an area and should they be removed? There is one fairly large one under my left arm that my bra does irritate at times.

A: These ugly brown spots, which my chief of dermatology used to call "barnacles on the ship of life," are real nuisances in the elderly. They scale, flake off, and itch horribly in some patients. Actually, since I treated *my* first one last year, I'll now refer to them as "spots due to wisdom and maturity." One dermatologist calls them "late-onset birthmarks" because the genes necessary to form them have always been there, but the spots don't appear until the necessary age is reached.

The real name for these crusty things is *seborrheic keratosis* (seb-o-REE-ick ker-a-TOE-sis). Classically, they have a waxy, stuck-on appearance, which has been likened to a drop of warm brown candle wax dropped on the skin. Often they have little dots on their surfaces, indicating areas where the keratin, or dead layer of the skin, has formed small plugs.

More numerous? I guess so! I've seen as many as several *hundred* of these flaky spots on a single patient. Often, as your history suggests, they do itch somewhat. Basically, though, they're harmless "gifts" from your ancestors; that is, they are inherited, and you're quite likely to pass them on to your progeny.

Seborrheic keratoses (SKs) are so widespread in our population that I've received literally hundreds of questions regarding them. In a television interview, I recently offered an informational sheet telling people about seborrheic keratosis, and the next day I received 400 individual inquiries about it. You can see what an incredibly common and annoying problem this is. The following is just one more example of how diverse the presentation of these spots can be.

Q: I am 74 years old. When I was 11 years old, I had smallpox. Over the past five years, I have developed two large, brown, crusty spots on my face in about the same place that I had scars from the smallpox. These spots are about the size of a fingernail, and my family doctor told me to leave them alone. Is there anything I can do? Were they caused by the smallpox scars being there?

A: The appearance of these spots some fifty years after your smallpox makes it impossible that they had anything to do with the spots. Their appearance in and around the old smallpox scars is purely coincidental.

Unfortunately, family physicians often *do* say to leave them alone, but only until the doctors *themselves* get a few. Then they swarm into the offices of their dermatologist colleagues to have them removed. And this is partly understandable. They spend their whole day dealing with serious diseases; often, they don't realize how distressing a disfiguring spot on a person's face, neck, or back can be. And even if they did, they really don't have the tools to fix the spots without scarring.

This brings up the treatment of SKs. Ordinarily, we use cryosurgery (freezing with liquid nitrogen). Light freezing of the spot causes a microscopic blister to form under the keratosis. This dries up into a scablike crust, which falls off within two to three weeks.

DERMALERT

Treatment of seborrheic keratoses is amazingly simple and efficient. There is no need to cut them off; freezing removes them completely, and with hardly a mark.

Usually, no mark is left when the crusts fall off. Sometimes dark-complected patients have a small dark spot left in the area, but this should fade nicely with time. "Just think, Dr. Bark," said one elderly patient with virtually hundreds of SKs, "I'll be able to swim as fast as my kids when you get all these barnacles off!"

Q: I am obese and have a large number of small, light brown, "spongy" blemishes under my breasts. My doctor has told me that they are nonmalignant, and that they can be removed surgically. I am sure this would be very time-consuming, because of the number of them. I am not interested in them for cosmetic reasons, because I am 62 years old. But occasionally one or two spots become a little sore or bothersome if they are rubbed by clothing. If I scratch my scaly blotches with my fingernail hard enough, they'll actually come off. Will they stay off?

A: Probably not. The cells which make up the hard spot, or keratosis, are in the deep epidermis, and it's unlikely that you could scratch hard enough to remove them for good. However, a modification of your "fingernail surgery" has been developed, in which the dermatologist freezes the spots lightly, and then scrapes them off with a curved knife blade called a curette.

After this procedure, the patient actually leaves the office without the spot. The disadvantages of this cryocurretage method, as it is called, is that an occasional patient will be more disposed to develop hyperpigmentation, or pigment darkening after cryocurettage, than after straight cryosurgery without the scraping procedure. The patient's going to have a scab anyway, so why not let the freezing do the whole job? In addition, bleeding and scarring occur sometimes with the scraping technique.

Q: Will these things turn into cancer?

A: No, assuming that you've got the right diagnosis. However, one of my greatest friends said once, "Assume makes an ASS out of U and ME." So get them checked to make sure of the correct diagnosis. The fact is that seborrheic keratoses are neither sunlight-induced nor precancerous, if that is what they are.

DERMALERT

Seborrheic keratoses are not malignant, but let your dermatologist determine which lesions are really SKs.

Q: Why take them off, then?

A: Seborrheic keratoses slowly enlarge over the years, and even though you may not think that, from a cosmetic standpoint, they need to come off right now, you may in the future. So I usually advise patients to have the ones in potentially objectionable areas removed when they are small. It certainly makes the task easier.

Q: What about the ones that my surgeon just wants to cut off? Wouldn't that be good enough?

A: Not if you're interested in not having a scar in all those areas! Regular cutting surgery goes right through the thickness of the skin, causing a scar every time one of them is taken off. But cryosurgery makes a very "physiological" type of split right at the base of the epidermis, which doesn't scar.

DERMALERT

Don't have SKs surgically cut off.

Q: What about burning them off with the electric needle?

A: Much the same is true here, as far as scarring is concerned. If the current is very low in the electric needle, some of these lesions can be coaxed off without scarring, but this takes a very deft hand on the part of the surgeon.

Q: I have "moles" that started under my arms and spread to my back and now are spreading all over my body, including my head and neck. But now, the last straw, they're growing on my face. Are they, in fact, contagious?

A: SKs are not contagious. They have though, in the past, been spoken of as seborrheic "warts," and that's probably where that idea came from. Touching them, or someone who has them, is not going to cause them to appear.

DERMALERT

SKs are not contagious. They are not real warts.

Giving the Death Penalty to Skin Tags

Q: I am 67 years old and had never had any skin problems until two years ago, when several threadlike warts appeared around my neck. After they became larger and turned brownish in color, a dermatologist snipped them off, saying that they might grow back. They are now doing this. What are they and what can I do?

A: These small "string moles," as they are called, are made up of two different types of structures. One is a miniature SK, which we've just discussed. The other is a tiny outpouching of actual skin, called an *acrochordon*. String moles are a genetic condition and are more common in those who are overweight.

These lesions are noncontagious and nonmalignant, but they surely are one of the most annoying nuisances of the human skin. They constantly catch on dresses, sweaters, clothing, and necklaces. They're also a favorite target for babies, who'll grab anything in sight and try to twist them off. Ouch! That hurts!

Other favorite places for skin tags to develop are the armpits and the groin, where they tend to be somewhat bigger. These lesions definitely tend to be more numerous in people who are overweight. It seems, sometimes, that one needs not only the genes for them but the size as well.

Some time ago, researchers reported that skin tags were more likely to occur in diabetics, but the studies necessary to confirm this were apparently never done. It's very possible that, since they occur more often in the overweight individual, obesity is the reason we see more diabetes, too. In other words, obesity may be the cause of both conditions. Recently a study related them to polyps in the colon as well. So people with bowel symptoms *and* skin tags should be examined for these large bowel outgrowths too.

The best treatment is very gentle, delicate electrocution of the string mole with an electric needle. The current must be extremely low in order not to scar the skin underlying the skin tag. A few years ago I had a patient ask if they could be frozen off. She was very apprehensive about electricity, because she had had some removed that way several years before. "Look, I'll show you," she said, as she pulled down her turtle neck sweater, "just look at *this*!" She revealed tens and tens of BB-sized, whitish scars all over her neck!

"Looks like something was done here before," I said conservatively.

"Sure was," she admitted, "But what I'd like to know is, what kind of instrument did the doctor use, a branding iron?"

I showed her a few pictures of the way skin tag removal is

supposed to turn out, and she agreed to let me try a few on the side of her neck which had not been treated. She returned several weeks later with virtually no marks in the areas, and we treated hundreds more.

DERMALERT

String moles, or skin tags, can be very deftly removed so that no mark is left, with a tiny charge of electricity. Ask your dermatologist about it.

Q: I have a small growth, perhaps a wart, on my eyelid. Would a dermatologist like yourself be the type of doctor I should go to to have it removed?

A: A dermatologist should at least evaluate the lesion before anything is done, to make absolutely sure it's just a skin tag. There are virtually hundreds of lumps and bumps which can occur around the eyelids, and proper diagnosis is crucial. However, skin tags, or *papillomas*, as the eye surgeons (ophthalmologists) call them, are the most common by far.

If, indeed, it is a skin tag, then sparking the spot with an electric needle (again, on very low current) is a very logical way to take it off. The largest one of these papillomas, of which I have photos in my collection, was as big as a *large grape*, on the lower eyelid of one of my patients. It had been there so many years, that it had begun to evert, or turn down, the lower lid, so that his eye watered constantly. The tears finally made him seek treatment.

I froze the main body of this huge bump on two different occasions, and sparked off the rest with my trusty Electrocator, and he went home happy.

Q: I have little wart-looking things on my neck which have now spread pretty much all over my chest. Over the years, doctors have told me that they were caused by a virus and that after menopause, they would go away. Someone else said clothes rubbing the skin caused them. I have had them burned off with acid and electric needles and cut off, but they continue to multiply. Help!

A: This shows the depth of the misinformation on common problems like skin tags. That's exactly why I'm sitting here, slaving over a hot typewriter to correct all these crazy myths! Virus? Rubbish! Go away after menopause? Nonsense! And clothes rubbing the skin, as I've said, can irritate them, but not cause them.

The old-timers did have one saying that was at least therapeutically effective: Tie a horse hair around the little critters, and they'll fall off in a week. This method of strangulating the blood supply of skin tags is still used effectively by some. However, I think, as do most dermatologists, that something removed from the skin should always be sent in for examination by a pathologist.

Q: If you take small skin tags off my neck, will more come out because of that?

A: Dr. Marsh, my mentor in dermatology, has a favorite saying about the growth of new skin tags. "Joe, treating skin tags is like stamping out roaches," he says. "You kill one and ten come to the funeral!" While killing them off doesn't really make new ones appear, the tendency to have them does continue, and new ones grow constantly.

Out, Out Hand Spot!

Q: Recently my husband went to the doctor for black spots on the backs of his hands. The doctor said they were age spots and nothing could be done. But we saw what you did to a hand spot on television, and we would like to know if there is an over-the-counter medicine you can get for this condition.

A: These "birthday presents," as I like to call them, are usually flat, darkly pigmented brown spots on the backs of the hands. They're called "liver spots," because they were previously thought (incorrectly) to come from liver trouble.

Unfortunately, there are no lotions that will dependably remove them or make them lighter. The only way I know to do this effectively is through the use of cryosurgery. A light liquid nitrogen spray over the lesions will peel them off in one to three weeks, leaving a little red spot which will take a month or two to go away. The spots almost always turn back to normal skin color after a time, leaving you practically "spotless."

Q: Can liver spots on the *face* be removed with liquid oxygen, and is it successful?

A: Previously, in our area, liquid *nitrogen* wasn't available, but liquid *oxygen* was. So, since the cold of each is equally effective, dermatologists in this area used liquid oxygen for a long time. Shortly after I started practice, liquid nitrogen became the accepted standard.

DERMALERT

Liver spots on the hands and face can be removed easily with liquid nitrogen spray.

Yes, the age spots on your face can indeed be removed by cryosurgery, in most cases. A light spray is usually all that's needed. But remember, if any of your spots are red, scaly, or raised up above the surrounding skin, you should definitely have them checked by a dermatologist. They could be many different types of spots.

These facial, flat, fairly tan spots are sometimes called *actinic lentigo*, or "sun freckles," indicating their relationship to sun and a freckling tendency.

Q: Do they turn into cancer?

A: Some of the spots, called *actinic keratoses*, do. They are discussed in Chapter 17.

Q: I have heard you talk about a cover-up for birthmarks. Will it work on the brown spots that appear on the face in old age?

A: Yes, the Covermark system, mentioned in Chapter 3, should work for nonraised lesions. However, raised or not, they should be checked for a tendency to be premalignant and for the possibility that they'll come off much better by cryosurgery than by covering them up.

Red Bumps

Q: I would like to know about the tiny red spots above the skin similar to moles, which have appeared on me and my husband lately. They seem to be multiplying. Two of our three adult sons are beginning to get some too. Both sides of our families had numerous moles, and therefore we have them too, but I would like to know if these red dots are related.

A: These tiny reddish bumps are called *cherry angiomas* (De Morgan's spots). They are another benign sign of TMB, composed of hundreds of dilated (wide-open) capillaries in the skin surface. They indeed do arise more frequently in families with a history of them, and the chances of you passing these lesions on to your kids is excellent.

DERMALERT

Cherry angiomas (De Morgan's spots) can be eliminated beautifully with an electric needle.

Note carefully that these lesions do not ordinarily bleed, unless they have occurred in an area of trauma, such as the shaving areas. But if they are nicked and start to bleed, they're tough to stop. They also slowly enlarge with time. I've seen ones as big as an eraser by the hundreds on patients' chests.

Although from a medical standpoint they really don't need to be treated, patients often want them off for cosmetic reasons. In that case, we haul out the Electrocator again, and zap them with a tiny current from its electric needle. They'll usually go away without a trace after this procedure.

Varicose Veins of the Skin

Q: I've got a bluish spot on my ear that looks like a blood spot under the skin, but it doesn't go away. If I press on it, the blue leaves for a few seconds. Have I got cancer?

A: I doubt it. Your description fits that of a spot we call a "venous lake." These bumps are sometimes called *varicose* (enlarged) *veins* of the skin. They're not cancer and they won't turn into cancer. Your dermatologist can remove them with a simple minor surgical procedure. These spots are quite similar to the ones historically called "caviar spots" on the undersurface of the tongue. These buckshotlike bumps get slowly more numerous with age. Most of us will have some of them at some time but they're harmless. Look under your tongue to see if you have them already. It'll give you some idea of how many TMBs you've suffered.

Bruising

Q: I am 70 years old and very easily get black-and-blue marks on my arms. Does this mean I have problems with my blood? Just the slightest bump seems to cause one.

A: These spots, previously called *senile purpura* (a horrible term), are now referred to as *ecchymoses* (eck-ee-MO-sees), or superficial bruises. There are several reasons why we tend to get these when we grow older. First and foremost, the skin thins as aging occurs, causing the strong support network of collagen in the skin to weaken. This weakening allows the tiny blood vessels in the upper skin layers to break at the slightest tap, just as you describe. Also, sunlight seems to play a part in the weakening of these vessels. They seem to be much more common in sun-exposed people than in others.

There is no real way to prevent ecchymoses from happening. The only way I've been able to help patients with them is to advise the person to be extraordinarily careful about trauma on their arms. And if they do see one developing after a minor injury, keep firm pressure on the exact spot where the injury took place for about five to seven minutes. This allows the blood to clot in the wall of the injured blood vessel, stopping further leakage. At least the pressure technique can prevent them from getting too large.

DERMALERT

Treatment for bruising on the arms of the elderly is *prevention*. The arms should be shielded from any possible minor trauma. If an injury occurs, put firm pressure on the spot for five to seven minutes.

One more important fact about ecchymoses—the chronic, repeated deposition of blood under the skin will often leave a brownish discoloration in the skin substance itself. That's why it's important to try to *prevent* these lesions. Use my "firm pressure" method, and you'll see results.

The fact that you get ecchymoses in your seventies does not necessarily mean that you have a blood disease. However, any serious bleeding tendency, especially if not localized to the arms, should be evaluated by your doctor. He or she may want to do clotting tests and other tests on your blood and look for internal diseases.

One other thing you might try for your bruising problem. Dermatologists writing in the November 1985 *Schoch Letter* (a newsletter for dermatologists) say that a vitamin with zinc, called Vi-Zac, taken twice daily, can dramatically help the problem.

They also caution that people with the problem should not take any aspirin unless directed to do so for some other medical problem. Aspirin causes easy bruising by stopping the aggregation of the body's platelets, an essential clotting factor.

Q: I have what I think may be a slightly different problem. My bleeding areas under the skin are beginning to cause scars in the skin. You haven't mentioned this, and I'm wondering if I have something different?

A: You've got the extremely fragile skin I've just described, plus, from time to time you've had actual tears in the skin, leaving scars behind to heal with these whitish discolorations. A lot of older people get these, quite innocently, when they apply tape to their arms. The simple removal of the tape can cause a serious rip in the delicate skin of the arms. *Never* apply adhesive tape to the arms of the elderly, if it can be avoided. All bandages needed in the area of the thin skin of the arms should be *wrapped* gently with gauze bandages.

Q: I am a 57-year-old housewife, and I have tiny bruises about the size of a pinpoint, which my doctors have called *petechiae*, all over my body, thighs, and arms. They've been present for years. I now have ten to fifteen per square inch, and I keep getting more all the time. Some seem to get a little larger. My doctor has taken a blood test and says petechiae are nothing to be concerned about. I've never seen this problem discussed anywhere. Can you give me any info on the subject?

A: Petechiae, if that's indeed what you've got, are tiny blood hemorrhages in the very uppermost layer of the skin. There is a variety of causes, from just being normal to having leukemia or lymphoma. Apparently, your doctor has thoroughly ruled out serious medical diseases, but he or she may choose to send off a skin biopsy to see, on a microscopic level, what's actually going on in the skin. Sometimes various irritations of the blood vessels, called *vasculitis*, can be found in this manner. Then the exact causes of the vasculitis must be sought with detailed testing. It's not only the elderly who get petechiae, so anyone with red spots should get them looked at.

Snow on the Roof

Q: My hair is turning gray, and I'm only 38. I think that's really too young for a man to have gray hair. How safe is Grecian Formula to use?

A: Grecian Formula is a gradual coloring agent which contains the chemical lead acetate. The chemical attaches to the hairs and does not reflect light very well. This makes the hair surface take on a black look. For years dermatologists have okayed these products as long as the manufacturer's directions are followed. I personally like gray hair. Although Grecian Formula is probably safe to use, I would definitely follow the package directions very carefully, and would be very careful to put it only on the hairs, and not on the skin. The real disadvantage is cosmetic—only various shadings of black can be produced, so men (or women, for that matter) with brown, red, or blond hair will find no use for the product.

Want a better idea? Why don't you try some of the color rinses and dye that women use? Their safety records are good, and the color selection is almost infinite. Or better yet, have a professional salon help you mask your gray. So easy, and much faster results, too!

Stasis Dermatitis—A Vein Problem, Not a Vain Problem

Q: I have a spotted, scaly, dark color on my ankle. My doctor says it is poor circulation, and to keep it moist with lotions and creams and be careful not to injure the skin. Can you suggest other treatments?

A: Your problem is probably *stasis dermatitis*, or irritated skin due to slowing of the circulation. This is an extremely common rash in men as they age, and also in women who have had previous vein operations.

The scaly, itchy rash begins because of the slowed blood flow to the leg skin, caused by atherosclerosis (hardening of the arteries), past vein problems, chronic heart failure, and so on. It's a troublesome disease, because we haven't yet figured out how to prevent problems in the circulatory system. Usually, we end up treating the disease after it has occurred.

I can't stress enough how much leg elevation means in trying to keep leg skin intact, once stasis dermatitis is discovered. Elevation of the heels to a point slightly higher than the hips, *without bending the knees*, is the best way to get the blood flowing better in the legs.

Q: Will support hose help my circulation?

A: If you obtain your support hose on your doctor's prescription, such as T.E.D. or Jobst brands, they will most assuredly help your blood flow better in your legs. I myself wear a special type of men's support dress socks. They're called Jobst Stride Stockings, and you can inquire about these very comfortable socks from:

The Jobst Institute
653 Miami Street
P.O. Box 653
Toledo, Ohio 43694

However, the conventional support hose which are available in department stores are not very effective because they are not custom-measured. They can't, therefore, help individual problem veins. The Jobst Institute, however, will custom-measure your leg so you'll get the greatest benefit from elastic stockings.

The other treatments used in stasis dermatitis are various creams containing enzymes, cortisones, and/or antibiotics.

Q: Will the dark color ever disappear?

A: The brownish-tan stain in the skin of your legs is caused by the deposition of iron in the skin from blood which has leaked out previously. This occurs each time a small injury occurs. It's much the same as the staining we discussed under ecchymoses. Some of the pigment is also melanin, the natural color material of the skin. This component of the dark skin color can lighten over time, but it does indeed take a long time.

Leg Ulcers

Q: I've got ulcers on my legs. What should I do?

A: Ulcers are the most dreaded complication of stasis dermatitis. They result not only from the inflammation of the skin but from the actual death of a patch of it.

Dealing with leg ulcers is one of the hardest tasks facing the dermatologist. Over the years, a hundred different remedies have been tried. We've used everything from twenty-four-karat gold leaf, to antibiotics, to *table sugar* packed into the ulcer, to creams, injections, and surgery. Many of these have been successful, and each of them has ardent physician supporters. However, there are two newer advances which show great promise.

The first is Debrisan, a new substance for healing the ulcer from the inside. Once into the ulcer, this material, called *dextranomer*, pulls in moisture, broken-down skin cells, bacteria, and other products of the healing process. The dextranomer beads soak up these substances, which are removed when the beads are washed out. When applied two or three times daily, a whistle-clean ulcer base can be achieved, allowing speedy healing to occur. If necessary, good skin can be grafted from another site to cover the open ulcer.

The second major new development in the healing therapy for ulcers is a material called OpSite. This is an adhesive film which is applied to the surface of the ulcer. The plastic-looking sheet is a so-called semipermeable membrane, which allows oxygen to pass into the healing area. The moisture, however, is held inside, allowing the skin cells to glide over the wound, healing over the defect much faster.

The material has to be applied in a very special manner, however, and a dermatologist needs to monitor the OpSite carefully to guard against a so-called "silent infection." If this occurs, bacteria can overrun the ulcer, preventing healing instead of encouraging it.

DERMALERT

New therapies for leg ulcers, such as Debrisan and OpSite, make it possible to heal them relatively quickly.

Regardless of which of the many useful treatments is chosen to heal your leg ulcer, it's important to get it healed. Chronic ulcers are a source of infection not only for the legs but for the rest of the body as well.

Shingles—A Herpesvirus

While ulcers are a tough problem for the elderly, there are, you'll find, none tougher than shingles.

Q: I had herpes six months ago which started as a pain in my shoulder, and I broke out in blisters all the way down my arm to the palm of my hand, on my fingers, and even under my fingernail. My doctor gave me some cortisone shots in the rump, several prescriptions for codeine, and put me on vitamins B and E. He even tried heat treatments to my back.

Then I went to see a neurologist who prescribed Ascriptin and later Naprosyn, neither of which have helped. He called my problem postherpes neuralgia. Please help! So far I've had two electromyograms, one electroencephalogram, one electrocardiogram, nine x-rays, seven treatments by a chiropractor, one blood count, two heat treatments, several dozen dope pills, and hundreds of aspirin, and I *still* have a no-account arm!

A: You've really found out about shingles the hard way! Let me start by commenting on your statement that you had "herpes." The virus which starts shingles actually *is* one of the herpes viruses. But it's only phylogenetically related to herpes simplex. That is, you don't catch shingles from sexual activity or herpes simplex from a shingles patient. Just thought I'd clear that up before we start to talk about shingles.

The virus that caused your shingles is called the *varicella-zoster virus* (VZV). All of you who are parents, and who have seen your children through all the typical childhood diseases, probably recognize varicella as chicken pox. Yep! That's right, chicken pox is the cause of shingles. Let me explain. Most of us have chicken pox as kids, it heals fine, and we think the disease is gone. But the virus actually goes into hiding in the nerve roots of the spinal cord, where it'll stay for the rest of our lives.

Later, VZV can be reactivated, only this time it doesn't produce a generalized case of chicken pox. Instead, a localized case of chicken pox-like blisters results from the virus invading the exact skin supplied by the nerve roots where it has hidden all these years. When the virus reaches the skin again, it starts to form blisters which are much worse than the childhood chicken pox.

Unlike chicken pox, shingles is a very painful disease, and usually affects adults middle-aged and older. I've often been called to the cardiac intensive care unit to see patients with chest pain and a strange rash. The severe chest pain frequently started several days earlier than the rash, causing the physician to suspect a serious heart attack. Naturally, we're always happy to see a one-sided stripe of blisters appear on the patient's chest, indicating that he or she hasn't really had a heart attack at all.

Amazingly, you are contagious while you have shingles—not for shingles but for chicken pox. A shingles patient never gives another person shingles, just chicken pox. So if you don't want members of your household to get chicken pox, then stay away from them when you have shingles.

DERMALERT

Shingles is really limited, adult onset chicken pox! If you have shingles, you can't give them to anyone, but you certainly are contagious for chicken pox.

You've certainly had the "route" as far as treatment goes. The pain relievers and cortisone shots are meant to decrease the pain, but they usually cannot get rid of it. Later we'll talk about advances in treating it. Vitamin therapy is useless.

All the tests you went through must have been tough, but I'll tell you why your doctor did them. He, and all of us for that matter, is concerned about the general health of patients with herpes zoster. That's because it's been shown and remarked about for years that those with an atypical course of zoster, such as spreading of the rash outside the usual bandlike area, are at some increased risk for cancer, usually of the digestive tract or lymph system. Remember the story of Paul in Chapter 1? It's in cases like these that we thank VZV for alerting us to such a problem.

Q: How often is cancer the problem which activates VZV?

A: It happens very rarely. In fact, some studies refute the claim that there's an association, but who could afford not to look? I personally study every VZV patient over 45. Usually, that amounts to getting at least a chest x-ray and blood count.

DERMALERT

In the elderly, the appearance of a really bad case of shingles can indicate the presence of an internal malignancy.

Q: Is shingles a nerve problem?

A: Not from the standpoint of being a "nervousness," that is, emotional, problem, but as far as the nervous system is concerned, the actual fibers of the nerves do carry and transmit the virus to the skin.

Q: I had a permanent and afterward I noticed a spot on my

forehead which was very red and felt like a sensitive burn. I washed this spot, but the burning lasted for about a week. The beauty operator thought she might have failed to put enough cotton around the hairline when she gave the permanent, but I shortly broke out in "shingles" and the initial breaking out took place in the exact spot where the perm burn occurred. Was there any relationship between the two?

A: VZV doesn't usually break out in simple areas of trauma, such as an irritation by permanent fluid. In that sense, your VZV attack is purely coincidence. But, like the cardiac intensive care unit stories, it shows how coincidence often points to a false cause. That's the exact mechanism through which folk tales start. You just happened to get shingles at the same time as your permanent.

Q: My husband has had shingles over two years now, and he has tried everything without getting any relief. He had them around his left ribs and up his back, and there are some that have not yet gone completely away. They are now little white scars on the chest skin.

The problem is that they ache and burn almost constantly, and nothing seems to give him any relief. Can you recommend something that would cool it off and relieve the pain?

A: You know how infrequently chicken pox scars? Well, when a patient gets VZV, he or she already has immunity to the virus in most cases. That's apparently why it just stays in one dermotome, or skin stripe. But the fact that immunity is present means that the reinfection is fought much harder by the body, resulting in a deeper mark in the spots where the blisters were. Most people who have had zoster do indeed have some scars, and this can be quite a problem if they appear on the face.

Treatment of his pain (called post-zoster neuralgia or PZN), as we've discussed, is extremely difficult. Chronic pain relievers are the only proven help, but dermatologists and neurologists are now trying other substances, such as antidepressants, Dilantin (phenytoin, a drug used for seizures), Taractan (chlorprothixine, a tranquilizer associated with decreased pain), and Haldol (haloperidol, a drug used in psychiatric disorders). At least it'd be worth a try asking your dermatologist how the trials of these drugs are progressing. As of this writing, they help some and don't help others.

In 1980, Japanese researchers reported that patients with the persistent pain of PZN were having significantly reduced symptoms after a technique called *cryocautery*. In cryocautery, the painful dermatome, or skin stripe, where the herpes zoster infection originally occurred is rubbed with dry ice, or sprayed with freon. This causes intense local pain, followed by the blistering we usually see after cryosurgery for warts and other benign diseases. The frozen places heal somewhat lighter than the surrounding areas, but when the treatments were continued for an average of eight treatments per patient at two- or three-week intervals, the pain subsided in all but one patient. This technique does indeed produce a blistering, second-degree freeze "burn," so it's necessary to be followed relatively closely while the treatments are progressing.

Patients with PZN are willing to go anywhere and try almost anything, but I'd caution you to try a medicine only after some testing has been carried out showing effectiveness.

Q: Can shingles affect the eye? I've heard several different stories about this.

A: You bet it can! One of the most dreaded complications of shingles on the face is that they might affect the cornea, or clear part, of the eye. They usually do this if the *tip of the nose* is affected and actually has had blisters on it. This means that the nasociliary branch nerve has been affected, and that's the important one which supplies the cornea. And if the shingle virus infects the cornea, you're in trouble! (Ophthalmologists use potent antiviral ointments for this.) Other than that, you shouldn't have to worry about corneal involvement, even if the lids are severely involved. But most of us will consult an ophthalmologist to check on the eye condition of patients with zoster around the lids, just to be safe.

DERMALERT

If your shingles blisters affect the *tip of your nose,* see an ophthalmologist (eye physician and surgeon) immediately.

Q: I had shingles on my forehead one time; right between my eyes, where there was a large lesion, the scab fell off and left a scar which looks like I had a ruby there which popped out! What can I do to cover that up?

A: These scars can be quite difficult to mask. I'd try filling the defect with the help of Covermark cosmetics (mentioned in Chapter 3). It's either that, or put your ruby back in!

Whiteheads in the Elderly

Q: My skin problem is what I would term "whiteheads." I seem to be getting more and more of them at age 67! However, I can extract them with a disinfected needle and a hair pin. Now whiteheads are coming in the cavity of my eyes in which I am afraid to use that crude method. Is there an ointment that would dissolve the things? What method would you recommend?

A: Actually, you didn't do too badly, doctor! (That's what I call patients who treat themselves.) But stop doing your own acne surgery. You can cause real damage, and possible infection, in the crucial area around the nose and eyes. Let your real doctor do this. Remember the saying, "A person who treats himself has a *fool* for a patient."

You appear to have a problem known as Favre-Racachout syndrome, also known as nodular elastoidosis with cysts and comedones. Sounds complicated, but it really does describe it well. The problem results from the loose skin (elastoidosis) which accompanies TMB and damage from years of sunlight exposure. Small blackheads (comedones) form all over the upper cheeks and eye areas (the orbits), which need a type of acne surgery, using tools similar to the ones you've used.

DERMALERT

Whiteheads and blackheads on the upper outer cheeks are a very common complication of TMB. A special type of "acne surgery" can eliminate these troublesome spots.

A face-lift usually helps the Favre-Racachout problem too. At least 60 percent of my patients with this problem have the loose eyelid skin which is just ripe for what the plastic surgeons call a *blepharoplasty*, or lid job. This is one of the neatest operations ever invented, and it can make you look years younger. Think about it!

Treatment of this blackhead condition centers around pushing out the whiteheads and trying to prevent them in the future. We use a little tool something like your hairpin, as a matter of fact. It's called a comedo (blackhead) extractor. The trick is knowing how to do the procedure so you don't injure yourself. It's for this reason that I wouldn't ask you to go down to the drugstore and buy yourself one of these gadgets. Have an expert, your dermatologist, do it.

By the way, this problem of whiteheads and blackheads around the eyes is one of the all-time most popular "Say doc" diseases. That's a condition discovered on a relative of an office patient as the patient leaves the room. Usually the patient leaves first and the relative hangs behind for a minioffice visit, and says, "Say doc, what do you suppose these white things are on my cheeks?"

Wrinkles—Collagen Treatments

Q: A common complaint of older women (and men, too) who are afraid of a face-lift, or cannot afford one is wrinkling around the mouth. There is supposed to be a method for filling the lines or wrinkles in with a new substance. Can you tell us about this?

A: Sure! The new stuff is an injectable form of collagen. That, as you remember, is what comprises the support network of the skin. The Collagen Corporation has refined a technique for injecting the components of skin into a defect or depressed spot, such as a forehead wrinkle, where the material actually reassembles itself into near-human collagen. It's FDA-approved and I've discussed it thoroughly in Chapter 8. The medicine's called Zyderm, and can work wonders for the women you mention.

On March 7, 1983, the Collagen Corporation released a special bulletin to physicians indicating that one patient out of the many thousands treated with collagen for forehead wrinkles had apparently lost sight in one eye from the accidental injection of collagen into a blood vessel in the area of the forehead. They have cautioned dermatologists to make doubly sure that they are not injecting into a blood vessel during the procedure.

Q: What is the difference between a dermabrasion and a chemical peel?

A: Dermabrasion is the superficial sanding off of the upper two layers of the facial skin. A chemical peel refers to an acid treatment of the same layers of the skin. Both procedures are done to alleviate scarring and minor wrinkles in the facial skin. (See the discussion of these procedures in Chapter 8, and talk to your dermatologist and/or plastic surgeon about obtaining the procedures, if they are warranted.)

Yellow Patches on the Lids

Q: I would like information concerning cholesterol deposits on the inside corners of my eyes. I have had them removed surgically at one time (very painful, by the way), and they returned in a very short time. I have been on a low-cholesterol diet for years and they are still here. Is there any way to get rid of them safely?

A: These spots are called *xanthelasma*. This word is derived from a Greek word meaning "yellow plate," which is exactly what they look like. They represent a minor collection of oil below the surface of the eyelid skin. In some patients, they signify high levels of fats in the blood, such as cholesterol and/or triglycerides. In fact, we usually check patients for these abnormalities prior to treating them.

DERMALERT

Yellow eyelid oil spots may indicate high blood fat levels. Treating this problem may decrease your susceptibility to heart attacks in the future.

Xanthelasma lesions can be treated in many ways, and it certainly looks like you've found out about some of them. Surgery does work to remove them, and just because yours came back does not mean that the operation was unsuccessful. It's the nature of these "oil slicks," as we call them, to recur, so don't be too surprised if they grow back after your next attempt at removal either.

Besides surgery, some dermatologists paint the spots with dilute trichloroacetic acid. This causes a scab to form over the spot, and over the next week or two the yellowish plaque dumps right out. Usually, this occurs without any scarring.

Electrosurgery, such as that used on the skin tags we talked so much about earlier in this chapter, can also be used with great success. Just remember that with any method of removal, recurrence is the rule rather than the exception.

You can see that with advancing years come a host of new skin problems. These problems make aging much more uncomfortable, if not downright miserable. The whole point of this chapter is that you really don't have to put up with all the skin problems that come with age. The proper surveillance by your dermatologist, combined with the simple advice contained in this chapter, can keep telltale TMBs to a minimum.

Just remember to consult your dermatologist when you start to see the signs we've discussed in this chapter. To do so will help make your skin a soft, beautiful, and smooth covering as the decades pass. This, in the words of Dr. Al Kligman, may make it possible to "Die young as late as possible!"

21

The Real Skin Secret
Is You!

Congratulations! Now you've got all the information in your grasp to help your skin live a long, wrinkle-free, healthy, and beautiful life—so use it! *You* are the real secret to your skin health. *You* can make it all happen, if you'll just follow a few simple tips to healthy skin.

During many of my talks for the American Cancer Society, people always ask, "How can I really give myself the 'best shot' at living without cancer?" It's a question which really sums up what everyone wants to know about a terrible menace. But that very useful question has been the basis around which I have constructed this book: "What are the *Skin Secrets* I need to know to keep my body's largest organ healthy and beautiful all my life?" *Note*: The question was not "What can my *doctor* do to keep my skin healthy?" We now live in a world where responsibility for *acting* on information is ours, once we have it.

Here are some vital rules you've learned in *Skin Secrets* to keep you healthy:

1. A *baby's skin* is extremely fragile—don't do anything to it that you don't find absolutely necessary. Use a mild soap, and don't put medicated lotions and creams on an infant unless specifically ordered to do so by your pediatrician or dermatologist.

2. When your children's *oil glands* end their long hibernation in puberty, watch them like a hawk! If you catch their acne process early, you may virtually save their social lives. Insist on a regular cleansing program with soap and water, and demand early dermatologic care for any child with an acne problem.

3. *Avoid sunlight*! It's the single worst influence your skin will ever undergo. Just ask the 600,000 or so people who develop skin cancers every year. And don't forget to consider yourself an active member of my Tan is Tacky Club. Use an SPF-15 sunscreen *whenever* you'll be exposed to the sun.

4. *In my opinion, tanning parlors are a public menace.* Remember that even the so-called safe new systems of tanning beds can apparently cause problems as severe as cataracts, premature aging, skin cancer, and even changes in the immune system. Avoid them. Don't physically fry your beautiful skin.

5. Got something growing on you? *Get it checked*! Review the signs and symptoms of skin cancer listed in Chapter 17 at every opportunity. Procrastinating can just allow benign lumps and bumps to get bigger and harder to remove. And for malignant problems of the skin, waiting too long can be fatal. Remember that skin cancers are *easily* cured if caught in time.

6. Finally, *get yourself and your family a dermatologist*. In the final analysis, your dermatologist is the professional who *best* knows how to diagnose and treat skin diseases—not the allergist, pediatrician, gynecologist, or internist—the dermatologist! Skin is a dermatologist's *life*! And with the vigilant help of your dermatologist, your skin will healthily last you all yours!

Trademarks

Below is a list of trademarks used in this book, together with the firms in whose names the trademarks have been registered.

Accutane	Roche
Allercreme	ALCON Labs
Almay	Almay, Inc.
Aquacare	Herbert
Aristocort	Lederle
Ascriptin	Rorer
Atarax	Roehrig
Bain de Soleil	Charles of the Ritz
Band-Aid	Johnson & Johnson
Basis	Beiersdorf
Borghese's Green Color Corrector Foundation	Princess Marcellas
Buf-Puf	Personal Care Products
Caldesene	Pennwalt
Carmol 10	Syntex
Cetaphil	Owen
Chap Stick 15	Robins
Clinique's 15-rated sunscreen	Clinique Cosmetics
Clinique's Pore Minimizer Makeup	Clinique Cosmetics
Complex 15	Baker/Cummins
Coppertone Supershade 15	Plough
Cortaid solution	Upjohn
Covermark cosmetics	Lydia O'Leary
Debrisan	Johnson & Johnson
Dermage system	Cosmedics Research Labs
Dermalab X5, Dermalab X5T	Derma Labs
Dermal gloves	George Glove Company
DHS Tar	Person & Covey
Dilantin	Parke-Davis
Dove	Lever Bros.
Drithocreme	American Dermal
Dritho-Scalp	American Dermal
Drysol	Person & Covey
Ear-Eze	H & A Enterprises
Eclipse Lip Protectant	Dorsey
Efudex	Roche
Electrocator	Slatham
Elizabeth Arden	Elizabeth Arden Corp.
Emulave	Cooper Dermatologicals
Enisyl	Person & Covey
Fisherman's Sunglasses	Orvis
Fungizone	Squibb
Grecian Formula	Combe, Inc.
Haldol	MacNeil
Halog solution	Squibb
Hard as Nails	Sally Hansen
Inderal	Ayerst
Iocon	ALCON Labs
Ionil Rinse	ALCON Labs
Ionil T Plus	ALCON Labs
Jobst Stride Stockings	Jobst
Kenalog spray	Squibb

Keralyt gel	Westwood
K-Y Jelly	Johnson & Johnson
Lac-Hydrin	Westwood
LactiCare	Stiefel
Lanoxin	Burroughs Wellcome
Lasan Pomade	Stiefel
'Lectric Shave	Williams'
Locon	ALCON Labs
Lonil Rinse	ALCON Labs
Lonil T Plus	ALCON Labs
Loprox	Hoechst
Lotrimin	Delbay
Lowila	Westwood
Lubriderm	Warner-Lambert
Magic Shave	BenShefta
Mauve line	Cosmetics Research Labs
Melanex	Neutrogena
Monistat	Cilag-Chemie
Mycelex	Miles Pharmaceuticals
Nair	Carter-Wallace
Naprosyn	Syntex
Neet	Whitehall
Neutrogena soap	Neutrogena Corp.
Nizoral	Janssen
Noir sunglasses	Elder
Nudit	Medtech
OpSite	Acme United Corp.
Oxsoralen	Elder
P&S lotion	Baker/Cummins
Pearl line	Dermage-Cosmetics Research
Pentrax	Rydell
Phacid	Baker/Cummins
Potaba	Glenwood
PreSun 15	Westwood
Q-tip	Chesebrough Ponds
Regaine	Upjohn
Retin-A cream	Johnson & Johnson
R.V. Paque	Elder
Small Miracle	Clairol
Solbar PF	Person & Covey
Spectazole	Ortho
Sundown 15	Johnson & Johnson
Super Glue	Hermetite Products
Surgex	Sween
Tagamet	Smith Kline & French
Taractan	Roche
Tavist	Sandoz
T.E.D. support hose	Kendall
Tinactin	Schering Corp.
Total Eclipse 15	Dorsey
Ultra Derm	Baker/Cummins
Ultra Mide	Baker/Cummins
Vaseline	Chesebrough Ponds
Vi-Zac	Glaxo
X-seb, X-seb-T	Baker/Cummins
Zovirax	Burroughs Wellcome
Zyplast	Collagen Corp.
Zyderm	Collagen Corp.

Index

Accutane (13-cis-retinoid) therapy for
   acne, 71–74
Acne, 49–79
  Accutane therapy for, 71–74
  antibiotics in treatment of, 50, 56,
    64–68
  attitude of patient and, 51–53
  benzoyl peroxide therapy for, 51, 72
  birth control pills and, 67–68
  chocolate and, 53–54
  cosmetics and, 59–62
  diet and, 53–54
  emotions and, 55
  healing time for, 55–56
  hormones and, 62–63
  induced by physical pressure, 57–59
  in older persons, 56–57
  period-related, 69–70
  Retin-A cream for, 51
  scalp, and hair loss, 128
  soaps and, 54
  sunlamps and, 108–109
  sunlight and, 74–75

Acne (*cont*):
  treatments for, 50–53
  triamcinolone injection therapy for,
    78–79
  x-ray therapy for, 76–77
  zinc therapy for, 77–78
Acne-scarred skin:
  dermabrasion for, 82–84
  restoring, 81–91
  treatment of back scars, 88–89
  Zyderm injectable collagen implants
    for, 84–91
Acrochordon, 285
Actinic cheilitis, 237–239
Actinic keratosis, 231–232
Actinic lentigo, 257–258, 288
Acyclovir (Zovirax) therapy for herpes,
   267–270
Age, thinning of hair, 121–122
Aging skin, 279–303
Allergic contact dermatitis:
  and ear canal treatment, 142
  poison ivy as, 43–47

Allergies:
  to antibacterial soaps, 249
  to antibiotics, 41, 76
  to artificial fingernail glues, 201
  to cortisone cream, 166
  to cosmetics, 165–167
  to Efudex, 233
  familial, and atopic eczema, 39
  and immunotherapy, in treatment of
    alopecia areata, 129–130
  to PABA, 246–247
  to Zyderm collagen implants, 90
Aloe vera, 163
Alopecia:
  androgenetic (male pattern bald-
    ness), 112–114
  traction, 122, 193–194
Alopecia areata, 115, 128–132
Alopecia totalis, 132
Alopecia universalis, 132
Anhidrotic ectodermal defect, congenital, 108
Antibiotics:
  for acne, 50, 56, 64–68
  allergies to, 41, 76
  for jock itch, 183
  for sunburn, 249
Antibodies, 166
Antihistamine therapy for psoriatic
  itching, 218–219
Argon laser therapy for port-wine
  stains, 15
Aristocort, excess hair growth from,
  136–137
Armpit itch, 184–185
Aspirin:
  and bruising problem, 291
  and sunburn, 248–249
Astringents, 162–163
Axillary hyperhidrosis, 104–106

Baby oil, 9
Baby powder, 8, 9
Bacterial folliculitis, 128
Baldness, 111–116

Baldness (cont.):
  area (alopecia areata), 115, 128–132
  male pattern, 112–114
  (See also Hair loss)
Basal cell carcinoma, 234–235
  characteristics of, 238
Bathing:
  and dry skin, 271–274
  and eczema, 38
  and psoriasis, 209
  (See also Soaps)
Bathing trunk nevus, 13
Beard(s), 186
Beard bumps (razor dermatitis), 190–
  191
Beeswax-urea method for toenail removal, 182
Benzoyl peroxide therapy for acne, 51,
  72
Birth control pills:
  and acne, 67–68
  and hair loss, 126–127
  and melasma, 146
Birthmarks, 11–19
  hairy, 12–13
Black dermographism, 164
Black skin, 189–195
Blackheads (comedones), 300–301
  nasal, 74
Blepharoplasty, 301
Blisters:
  foot, as fungus, 182–183
  genital herpes, 263, 264
  hand eczema, 171–172
  impetigo, 23
  poison ivy, 44, 45
  shingles, 295–298
  sunburn, 249
Blue nevus, 241
Body odor, 107–108
Breast skin cysts, 148
Bruising, 290–292
Buf-Puf:
  for beard bumps, 191
  for keratosis pilaris, 102
Buttocks herpes, 264–265

Café au lait spots, 12
Calamine lotion for poison ivy, 46
Callaway, J. Lamar, 39, 106
Cancer (*see* Skin cancer)
Canthaxanthins (tanning pills), 247–248
Cellulite, 157–158
Cheilitis, actinic, 237–239
Cherry angiomas (De Morgan's spots), 289
Chicken pox:
    scars of, punch excision of, 88
    and shingles, 296–297
Chocolate and acne, 53–54
Cimetidine (Tagamet) therapy for excessive facial hair, 132–133
Cold sores, 260–262
Collagen treatments:
    for acne-scarred skin, 84–91
    for wrinkles, 301–302
Comedones (blackheads), 300–301
Complex 15:
    for dry skin, 274–275
    for hand eczema, 173
    for keratosis pilaris, 102–103
    for psoriasis, 209
    for wrinkles, 170
Congenital anhidrotic ectodermal defect, 108
Congenital melanocytic nevi, 13, 255
Contact urticaria syndrome, 174
Corn(s), soft, 159–160
Cornrow hair loss, 193–194
Cornstarch powder, 8, 9
Cortisone therapy:
    for acne, 78–79
    for acne-scarred skin, 89
    for alopecia areata, 129
    for excess hair growth, 136–137
    for itchy neck, 175
    for keloid itch, 192–193
    for pityriasis alba, 102
    for psoriasis, 208, 210–211
    for PUPP, 150
    for strawberry marks, 18
    for sunburn, 248–249

Cosmetics:
    and acne, 59–62
    allergies to, 165–167
    Covermark system, 16–17, 60, 155
    Dermage system, 61–62
    eye, 160–162
    lipstick, 275–276
    Pore Minimizer Makeup, 156
    in prevention of skin cancer, 163, 275
Covermark makeup system, 16–17
    and acne, 60
    for vascular spiders, 155
Cryocautery for post-zoster neuralgia, 299
Cryosurgery:
    for actinic keratosis, 231–232
    for freckle removal, 158–159, 257
    for genital wart removal, 186
    for liver spots, 287–288
    for molluscum contagiosum, 23
    for seborrheic keratoses, 282, 284
    for squamous cell carcinoma, 237
    for strawberry marks, 18
    for warts, 28
Cyproterone therapy for male pattern baldness, 119–120
Cystic acne, 73–74, 78–79
Cysts, breast skin, 148

Dandruff, 139–143
Dead Sea Psoriasis Treatment Center, 219–220
Debrisan therapy for leg ulcers, 294–295
De Morgan's spots (cherry angiomas), 289
Depilatories for hair removal, 134–136
Dermabrasion:
    for acne-scarred skin, 82–84
    for wrinkles, 302
Dermage system cosmetics, 61–62
Dermatitis:
    allergic contact, poison ivy as, 43–47
    exfoliative, and psoriasis, 205
    photo-, 249–250

Dermatitis (*cont.*):
  razor, 190–191
  seborrheic, 140–143
  stasis, 293–294
Dermatologists as physicians, 1–3,
    256–257
  in diagnosis of internal disorders,
    149, 154, 199, 292, 297, 302
Dermatopathic lymphadenopathy, 59
Dextranomer therapy for leg ulcers,
    294–295
Diabetes and vascular spiders, 154
Diabetic foot care, 160
Diaper, selection of, 7–8
Diaper rash, 5–9
Diet and acne, 53–54
Dihydrotestosterone, 113
Dimethylglyoxime kit, 168
Dinitrochlorobenzene therapy for
    warts, 31
Disease states, skin disorders in diag-
    nosis of, 1–3, 149, 154, 199, 292,
    297, 302
Dove soap, 38, 273
Dry skin, 271–277
Drysol therapy for excess sweating,
    105–108
Dyshidrosis (hand eczema), 171–175
Dysplastic nevus syndrome, 242

Ear flakiness, 141–142
Ear psoriasis, 212
Ecchymoses (senile purpura), 290–292
Eczema, 37–41
  atopic, 37, 40
  hand (dyshidrosis), 171–175
  nummular, 276
  treating itch of, 40–41
Efudex (5-fluorouracil) therapy:
  for actinic keratosis, 232–233
  for facial warts, 34–35
Electrodesiccator therapy for spider
    veins, 152
Electrolysis, 134
Electrosurgery:
  for skin tags, 285–286

Electrosurgery (*cont.*):
  for xanthelasma, 303
Emotions:
  and acne, 55
  and excessive sweating, 104
  and psoriasis, 217–218
Endocrine gland problems:
  and acne, 63
  and new hair growth, 136
Epilation, 134–137
Epstein, Ernst, 190
Erythrasma, 183
Erythromycin therapy for acne, 67
Estradiol therapy for female pattern
    hair loss, 122
Exfoliative dermatitis, 205
Eye(s), dark circles under, 162
Eye infection, mascara and, 160–161
Eyeliner, application of, 161–162

Face-lift:
  and dermabrasion for acne, 83
  for Favre-Racachout syndrome,
    300–301
  for spider veins, 154
Facial warts, 34–35
Fat suction, 157–158
Favre-Racachout syndrome, 300–301
Female pattern hair loss, 121–122
Female skin, 145–177
Fiedler, George, 61
Fingernail(s), 197–202
  dots in, 202
  pits in, in psoriasis, 205
  ridges on, 198–199
  splitting of (onychoschizia), 200–201
Fingernail fungus, 181–183
Fingernail warts, 30–31
Fisher, Alexander, 45
Flaky ears, 141–142
Fluorinated steroids, 153–154
5-Fluorouracil (Efudex) therapy:
  for actinic keratosis, 232–233
  for facial warts, 34–35
Folliculitis, bacterial, 128
Food facials, 170–171

Footwear, 159, 199
Formalin and salicylic acid therapy
    for plantar warts, 32–34
Freckles, 158–159
    sun, 257–258

Genital herpes simplex, 263–264
Genital warts, 177
Gentian violet therapy for flaky ears,
    142
Goldman, Leon, 15
Graham, Gloria, 61
Graying hair, 292–293
Grenz ray therapy for seborrheic der-
    matitis, 141
Griseofulvin therapy for tinea, 181

Hair, 111–137
    excessive, 132–137
    graying, 292–293
    growth cycle of, 125–126
    proper care of, 121, 123–124
Hair analysis, 117–118
Hair dandruff, 139–143
Hair loss:
    birth control pills and, 126–127
    cornrow, 193–194
    cyproterone therapy for, 119–120
    daily washing for preventing, 121
    female pattern, 121–122
    headgear, 117
    massage therapy for, 118
    minoxidil (Regaine) therapy for,
        118–119, 121, 122
    pregnancy and, 125–126
    progesterone therapy for, 120–121
    scalp acne and, 128
    (See also Alopecia; Baldness)
Hair removal creams, 134–135
Hair restorers, 115
Hair thinning:
    age related, 121–122
    in children, 122–123
    propranolol and, 127
    vitamins and, 114–115
    wheat germ shampoo and, 114–115

Hair transplants, 116
Hairy birthmarks, 12–13
Halo nevus, 253–254
Halog solution therapy:
    for ear canal psoriasis, 212
    for ear canal rashes, 142
Hand eczema (dyshidrosis), 171–175
Hashimoto, Ken, 190
Head lice, 96–97
Headgear and acne, 58–59
Headgear hair loss, 117
Heels, rough, 176–177
Heredity:
    in acne, 70
    in atopic eczema, 37, 39
    in dry skin, 276
    in keloid formation, 192
    in keratosis pilaris, 102–103
    in male pattern baldness, 113
    in melanoma, 242–243
    in psoriasis, 206–207
    in trichorrhexis nodosa, 123
Herpes, 259–270
    trauma and, 265
Herpes simplex virus, 259, 261
    genital type II, 263–264
Hodgkin's disease and shingles, 1–2
Hormones:
    and acne, 62–63
    and hair loss, 120–122
    and spider veins, 151
Hydrocortisone cream therapy:
    for eczema, 39, 40
    for poison ivy, 46
Hyperhidrosis, axillary, 104–106
Hypermelanosis, 194–195
Hypertropic scars:
    of acne, 88–89
    minor keloids as, 191

Immunotherapy for alopecia areata, 130
Impetigo, 23–24
Infantile psoriasis, 220
Infections, skin, 21–35
Injection therapy for leg spiders,
    155–156

Itching:
  armpits itch, 184–185
  from dry skin, 271–277
  from eczema, 40–41
  jock itch, 183–184
  in keloid formation, 192–193
  from lice, 93–94
  modified "scratch" for application
      of medicine, 40, 175–176, 210
  from poison ivy, 45–46
  from psoriasis, 210, 212, 218–219
  from PUPP, 150
  from scabies, 97–99
  from seborrheic keratosis, 281
  in skin cancer, 229–230
  from vaginitis, 66
Itchy neck, 176–176

Jewelry and nickel allergy, 167–170
Jock itch, 183–184

Keloids, 191–193
Kenalog spray for nickel allergy, 168
Keratin, 181
Keratosis:
  actinic, 231–232
  seborrheic, 281–284
Keratosis pilaris, 102–104
  inflammatory, 103
Ketoconazole (Nizoral) therapy for
      tinea versicolor, 100–101
Kligman, Albert M., 53, 61, 72
Koebner reaction in psoriasis, 210,
      211, 216, 218

Laser beam therapy:
  for leg spiders, 155
  for rosacea, 152–153
  for tattoos, 187–188
  for warts, 186
Lecithin, 274
Leg spiders, 154–156
Leg ulcers, 294–295
Lentigo maligna, 255
Lice:
  head, 96–97

Lice (cont.):
  pubic, 93–96
Lichen simplex chronicus, 175–176
Lindane shampoo therapy for lice, 94–97
Lipstick, 275–276
Liquid nitrogen freezing treatments
      (see Cryosurgery)
Liver spots, 287–288
Low pH shampoo therapy for sebor-
      rheic dermatitis, 141
Lubritz, Rachel, 61
Lymphadenopathy, dermatopathic, 59
Lymphocytes and allergies, 166
L-Lysine therapy for herpes, 265–267

Makeup (see Cosmetics)
Male pattern baldness (androgenetic
      alopecia), 112–114
Male skin, 179–188
Marsh, Glenn, xi, 75, 139
Mascara, eye infections from, 160–161
Mask of pregnancy (melasma), 146
Massage therapy for hair loss, 118
Medicines, over-the-counter and pre-
      scription compared, 3–4
Melanex therapy:
  for hypermelanosis, 194
  for pigment brown spots, 147
Melanin, 189, 240, 280
Melanoma, 239–243
  bathing trunk nevus and, 13
  characteristics of, 251
Melasma (pigment brown spots),
      146–148
Methotrexate therapy for psoriasis,
      215–216
Minocycline therapy for acne, 65
  tooth staining in, 69
Minoxidil (Regaine) therapy for hair
      loss, 118–119, 121, 122, 131
Mohs' microscopically controlled ex-
      cision, 235
Moisturizers:
  for dry skin, 274–275
  for eczema, 38–39
  for hand eczema, 173

Moisturizers (*cont.*):
  for keratosis pilaris, 102–103
  for psoriasis, 209
  and wrinkles, 170
Mole(s), 250–256
  characteristics of, 251
  hairy, 12–13
  string, 285
  traumatized, 186–187, 252
  (*See also* Nevi)
Molluscum contagiosum, 21–23
Moniliasis, 183

Nail(s) (*see* Fingernails)
Nail fungus, 181–183
Nephritis, impetigo and, 24
Neuralgia, post-zoster, 298–299
Neurodermatitis, 175
Nevus(i):
  bathing trunk, 13
  blue, 241
  congenital melanocytic, 13, 255
  Sutton's (halo), 253–254
  (*See also* Moles)
Nevus flammeus (port-wine stain),
  14–16
  Covermark makeup system for,
  16–17
Nickel allergies, 167–170
Nizoral (ketoconazole) therapy for
  tinea versicolor, 100–101
Nose:
  blackheads on, 74
  red, 152–153
Nummular eczema, 276

O'Leary, Lydia, 16
Onychoschizia, 200–201
OpSite therapy for leg ulcers, 295
Orentreich, Norman, 114
Oxsoralen, 130, 247–248
Ozone layer, 226, 241

PABA allergy, 246–247
Palmoplantar psoriasis, 212–213
Papillomas (skin tags), 284–287

Peck, Gary L., 68, 71
Penile psoriatic plaques, 216–217
Penile warts, 185–186
Petechiae, 292
Photodermatitis, 249–250
Pigment brown spots (melasma),
  146–148
Pinch test, 280–281
Pityriasis alba (sun spots), 101–102,
  231–232
Plantar warts, 31–34
Podophyllin therapy for plantar
  warts, 32–33
Poison ivy, 43–47
Poison ivy resin therapy for warts, 31
Pores, enlarged, 156
Port-wine stains (nevus flammeus),
  14–16
  Covermark makeup system for,
  16–17
Pregnancy:
  and acne treatment, 73
  and hair loss, 125–126
  and melasma, 146
  and psoriasis treatment, 213–214
  and spider veins, 151
  and stretch marks, 149–151
Primary irritant reaction, 174
Progesterone therapy for hair loss,
  120–121
Propionibacterium acnes, lipase from, 50
Propionibacterium minutissimum, 183
Propranolol and hair thinning, 127
Propylene glycol therapy for tinea
  versicolor, 100
Pruritic urticarial papules and plaques
  of pregnancy (PUPPP), 150–151
Pseudofolliculitis barbae (razor dermatitis), 190–191
Psoralen, 213–214, 248
Psoriasis, 203–221
  costs of treatment for, 214–215
  Dead Sea treatment for, 219–220
  ear, 212
  genetic basis of, 206–207
  in history, 220–221

Psoriasis (*cont.*):
    infantile, 220
    itching of, 210, 212, 218–219
    methotrexate therapy for, 215–216
    nutrition and, 207–208
    palmoplantar, 212–213
    penile plaques, 216–217
    PUVA therapy for, 212–214
    scaling in, 204–205
    scalp, 209–211
    stress and, 217–218
    treatment of, 208–220
Pubic lice, 93–96
Punch excision of chicken pox scars, 88
PUPPP (pruritic urticarial papules and plaques of pregnancy), 150–151
PUVA therapy:
    for alopecia areata, 130–131
    for psoriasis, 212–214

Razor dermatitis (beard bumps), 190–191
Red bumps, 289
Red face from fluorinated steroids, 153–154
Red nose, 152–153
Regaine (minoxidil) therapy for hair loss, 118–119, 121, 122, 131
Retin-A and benzoyl peroxide for beard bumps, 191
Retin-A cream therapy for acne, 51, 72
13-cis-Retinoid (Accutane) therapy for acne, 71–74
Ringworm (tinea corporis), 184
Rosacea, 152–153

Scabies, 97–99
Scalp acne and hair loss, 128
Scalp psoriasis, 209–211
Scalp reduction operation, 116
Seborrhea, 139
Seborrheic dermatitis, 140–141
    treatments for, 141–143

Seborrheic keratoses, 281–284
Selenium sulfide therapy for tinea versicolor, 100
Senile purpura (ecchymoses), 290–292
Shave, curettage, and electrodesiccation method, 236–237
Shave biopsy technique for moles, 252–253
Shaving, 186–187
    and beard bumps, 190–191
Shelley, Walter, 105
Shingles, 295–300
    Hodgkin's disease and, 1–2
Silver nitrate discoloration, 12
Skin cancer, 223–258
    cosmetics preventing, 163
    itching in, 229–230
    racial type and, 189–190, 227–228
    warts and, 26–27
    (*See also specific forms of skin cancer; e.g.,* Basal cell carcinoma; Melanoma; Squamous cell carcinoma)
Skin planing (*see* Dermabrasion)
Skin tags, 284–287
Smoking and wrinkles, 171
Soaps:
    and acne, 54
    and diaper rash, 8
    and dry skin, 272–273
    and eczema, 38
    and hand eczema, 172–173
    and photodermatitis, 249
    and poison ivy, 44
Sole (plantar) warts, 31–34
Spider veins, 151–154
    on legs, 154–156
Spironolactone therapy for excessive facial hair, 132–133
Squamous cell carcinoma, 235–239
    characteristics of, 238
Squaric acid dibutylester therapy for warts, 31
Stasis dermatitis, 293–294
Strawberry marks, 17–19

Stress:
  and acne, 55
  and excessive sweating, 104
  and psoriasis, 217–218
Stretch marks (striae), pregnancy
  and, 149–151
String moles, 285
Sulfa drugs, 75–76
Sulfur as drying agent, 76
Sun freckles, 257–258
Sun spots (pityriasis alba), 101–102,
  231–232
Sunburn, 248–250
Sunglasses, 250
Sunlamps, acne from, 108–109
Sunlight:
  and acne, 74–75
  and eczema, 41
  and Efudex reaction, 233
  and herpes sores, 261
  and melasma, 148
  and Retin-A, 51
  and skin, 225–230
  and wrinkles, 227–228
  and Zyderm injectable collagen im-
    plant, 90
Sunscreens, 243–246
  for melasma, 148
  for pityriasis alba, 102
Sutton's nevus, 253–254
Sweating:
  excessive underarm (axillary hyper-
    hidrosis), 104–106
  lack of, 108
Swimmers, sunscreens for, 245–246

Tagamet (cimetidine) therapy for ex-
  cessive facial hair, 132–133
Tanning beds, 224–225
Tanning pills, 247–248
Tanning salons, 224
Tar derivatives, 219
Tar shampoo, 211
Tattoos, 187–188
Teeth, antibiotic therapy for acne
  and, 68–69

Telogen effluvium, 125
Tetracycline therapy for acne, 50, 63–
  69
  and birth control pills, 67–68
  dental problems with, 68–69
  vaginitis as side effect of, 66–67
Tinea, 180–181
Tinea corporis (ringworm), 184
Tinea cruris, 183
Tinea versicolor, 99–101
Toenail fungus, 181–183
Topical antibiotics, allergies from, 41
Traction alopecia, 122, 193–194
Triamcinolone therapy:
  for acne, 78–79
  for alopecia areata, 129
Trichomycosis axillaris, 184–185
Trichorrhexis nodosa, 123
Two-foot-one-hand disease (tinea),
  180–181
Tylosis, 176–177

Ulcers, leg, 294–295

Vaginal warts, 177
Vaginitis, tetracycline therapy for
  acne and, 66–67
Varicella-zoster virus, 296–298
Varicose veins, 289–290
Vascular spiders, 151–154
  on legs, 154–156
Vasculitis, 292
Venereal diseases, 263–270
Venereal warts, 185
Verruca vulgaris (see Warts)
Viral warts, 177
Vitamin(s):
  hair thinning and, 114
  with zinc (Vi-Zac), for bruising
    problem, 291
Vitamin A and Accutane therapy for
  acne, 72–73
Vitamin B for fever blisters, 262
Vitamin D, 225
Vitamin E:
  and psoriasis, 208

Vitamin E (*cont.*):
  as "therapy" for warts, 29

Warts, 24–35
  and cancer, 26–27
  characteristics of, 251
  facial, 34–35
  fingernail, 30–31
  genital, 177
  penile, 185–186
  plantar, 31–34
  treatments for, 27–35
Weiss, Virginia, 131
Wheat germ shampoo and hair thin-
    ning, 114–115
Wheeler, Warren, 6
Whiteheads, 300–301
Winter itch, 271–277
Winter poison ivy, 47
Wood's light:
  for jock itch diagnosis, 183
  for pigment type determination,
    147

Wrinkles:
  collagen treatments for, 301–302
  moisturizers and, 170
  smoking and, 171
  sunlight and 227–228

X-ray therapy:
  for acne, 76–77
  for plantar warts, 32
  soft x-rays (Grenz rays) for sebor-
    rheic dermatitis, 141
Xanthelasma, 302–303
Xerosis, 272–273, 276

Yellow patches on lids (xanthelasma),
  302–303

Zaias, Nardo, 200
Zinc therapy for acne, 77–78
Zovirax (acyclovir) therapy for
  herpes, 267–270
Zyderm injectable collagen implants
  for acne-scarred skin, 84–91

To: SKIN SECRETS
Joseph P. Bark, M.D.
1401 Harrodsburg Road
Suite A-500
Lexington, KY 40504

If you have a skin question(s) for Dr. Bark, please fill out, detach, and mail this form.

Age_____Location of Problem_____Duration_____

Sex_____

Name_____

Address_____

City_____State_____Zip_____

YOUR SKIN QUESTION(S):

_____

_____

_____

_____

_____

_____

_____